"Nutrition is a proven key to success in endurance sports yet the correct approach is often neglected or misunderstood—and the consequences can be devastating to both performance and health. It is extremely refreshing to see the applications of years of sound sports nutrition research spelled out in a precise, comprehensive, and easy-to-read fashion. *The New Rules of Marathon and Half-Marathon Nutrition* is a must-read for beginner and elite-level runners."

—Kimberly Mueller, MS, RD, CSSD, sports dietitian, owner of
Fuel Factor Nutrition Coaching, and elite marathoner

"Finally, a short-cut to avoiding the wall! Matt Fitzgerald has the recipe for fueling for a peak performance. All runners will find this book informative and enlightening with advice that will immediately make a difference in training as well as racing."

—Greg McMillan, renowned running coach
and creator of the McMillan Running Calculator

"I highly recommend reading *Racing Weight* even if you don't need to lose any excess poundage. You'll come away with a better understanding of your physiology and also of food."

—Joe Friel, founder of TrainingBible Coaching and author of *The Triathlete's Training Bible* and *The Cyclist's Training Bible*

"*Racing Weight* answers the difficult questions athletes often have about dieting, including how to handle the off-season. The book gives readers a scientifically backed system to discover your optimum race weight, as well as five steps to achieve it."

—*Triathlete* magazine

"Reaching an ideal weight for endurance sports is important, but doing it the right way is even more important. Matt Fitzgerald provides scientific and sound advice for anyone trying to achieve their racing weight."

—Scott Jurek, author of *Eat and Run*, seven-time winner of the Western States Endurance Run, and two-time winner of the Badwater Ultramarathon

"Fitzgerald is a fountain of information on current research studies and findings from the sciences of healthy nutrition and exercise performance."

—*Ultrarunning* magazine

"Even if you are already a lean machine, you'll likely still learn something from *Racing Weight*. From how to determine your optimum weight, to improving your diet and training around it, to controlling your appetite and making your own fuel—it's all in this book."

—BikeRadar

"The mysteries of weight and its relationship to performance are unlocked in Matt Fitzgerald's *Racing Weight*. If you've got a basic handle on both training and nutrition, this book offers the means to improve both your diet and athletic performance."

—DailyPeloton.com

"Fitzgerald is going to go down as one of the most competent and prolific authors of books for serious runners covering just about every legitimate aspect of the all-important runner's lifestyle."

—Letsrun.com

"It's not too hard to convince cyclists that they can improve their performance if they drop their weight to an optimum level. However, that's generally as useful as a physician telling a client they need to lose weight and then sending them out the office door. There are endless diet or nutrition books out there, but very few specifically catering to the endurance athlete. Into this void comes *Racing Weight* by Matt Fitzgerald."

—Pezcyclingnews.com

The NEW RULES of
MARATHON and HALF-MARATHON
NUTRITION

ALSO BY **MATT FITZGERALD**

Iron War

Racing Weight

Brain Training for Runners

Performance Nutrition for Runners

The *NEW RULES* of
MARATHON and **HALF-MARATHON**
NUTRITION

A CUTTING-EDGE PLAN TO
FUEL YOUR BODY BEYOND
"THE WALL"

Matt Fitzgerald

Da Capo
LIFE
LONG

A Member of the Perseus Books Group

Designed by Pauline Brown
Set in 11.5 point Goudy Old Style Std by the Perseus Books Group

Library of Congress Cataloging-in-Publication Data

Fitzgerald, Matt.
    The new rules of marathon and half-marathon nutrition : a cutting-edge plan
to fuel your body beyond "the wall" / Matt Fitzgerald.
        p.   cm.
    Includes index.
    ISBN 978-0-7382-1645-4 (pbk. : alk. paper)—ISBN 978-0-7382-1646-1 (e-book)
    1. Marathon running—Training. 2. Runners (Sports)—Nutrition. I. Title.
GV1065.17.T73F57   2013
796.42'52071—dc23

                                                                    2012042839

First Da Capo Press edition 2013

Published by Da Capo Press
A Member of the Perseus Books Group
www.dacapopress.com

Da Capo Press books are available at special discounts for bulk purchases in the
U.S. by corporations, institutions, and other organizations. For more information,
please contact the Special Markets Department at the Perseus Books Group, 2300
Chestnut Street, Suite 200, Philadelphia, PA, 19103, or call (800) 810-4145, ext.
5000, or e-mail special.markets@perseusbooks.com.

LSC-C
10 9

CONTENTS

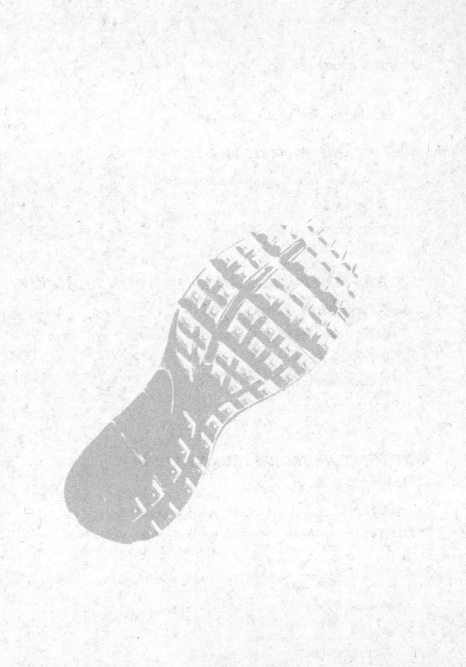

FOREWORD

BY KARA GOUCHER, ELITE RUNNER,
TWO-TIME OLYMPIAN AND FOUR-TIME NATIONAL CHAMPION

I hit the wall pretty hard in my first marathon. It was the 2008 ING New York City Marathon and I thought I was ready for it. The previous year I had won my first half marathon, beating marathon world record holder Paula Radcliffe in the process. My training for New York had gone really well. But less than 16 miles into the race my calves started to hurt, and things only got worse from there.

By the 20-mile mark the pain in my legs had climbed all the way up to my hips. When I finally reached Central Park, less than 2 miles from the finish line, I was ready to quit. I even looked for a place where I could pull off the course discreetly, but there were too many spectators, so I kept going.

When I crossed the finish line my first thought was that the race had been a total disaster, even though my third-place finish was the best by an American woman in the New York City Marathon since 1983, and my time of 2:25:53 was the fastest debut marathon ever by an American woman.

My second thought was that I couldn't wait to run another marathon.

That's the marathon for you. No matter who you are, your first marathon is bound to be the hardest thing you've ever done, but it hooks you. As soon as you finish it you can think of a dozen mistakes you made before the race and during the race, and you just know that if you fix them you can avoid hitting the wall the next time. There's something about the marathon that makes you want to master it.

Some of the biggest mistakes I made in my first marathon were nutritional. I hadn't done enough drinking practice in my training and as a result I dropped some of my bottles during the race and became dehydrated. I also hadn't done the homework necessary to find a sports drink that worked with my sensitive stomach, so what I was able to swallow did not sit well and became a painful distraction from the task at hand.

I worked on these issues and a few others and it paid off. I came nine seconds away from winning the 2009 Boston Marathon and I qualified for the 2012 Olympic Marathon. I couldn't have done these things if I hadn't gotten help along the way from sports nutrition experts including Matt Fitzgerald. When Nutrilite became my new nutrition sponsor I went to Matt for his opinion on its ROC2O sports drink. He checked it out for me and gave it a thumbs-up. I used it in the 2011 Boston Marathon, had no stomach issues, and ran a PR of 2:24:52 that made me the fourth-fastest American marathoner of all time.

I trust Matt's opinion on nutrition because it's always based on a combination of science, real-world experience, and practicality. This approach isn't as common as you might think. There's a lot of bad information floating around out there!

That's why I'm so happy that Matt has written *The New Rules of Marathon and Half-Marathon Nutrition*. Nutrition plays such a huge role in the marathon and also the half marathon, and now runners have somewhere they can turn to learn everything they need to know to fuel their bodies beyond the wall in these longer races.

I love the comprehensive approach that Matt has taken to this important subject. He covers everything from eating to reach your ideal racing weight to developing your own custom race nutrition plan, from the best meals and snacks for marathon and half-marathon training to nutrition on race morning. Then he bundles it all together in combined nutrition-training plans (what a great idea!) that make the whole process incredibly simple.

What's also great about *The New Rules of Marathon and Half-Marathon Nutrition* is its focus on the most cutting-edge information and practices. I still haven't run the best marathon I'm capable of and I believe that getting where I want to go as a marathoner will require that I keep learning and trying new things. I learned a lot from this book and I can't wait to see how I benefit from it, as I know you will, too.

THE WALL-HITTERS CLUB

My first marathon was the 1999 California International Marathon in Sacramento, California. I trained fairly seriously for it—up to 60 miles a week—and set an ambitious goal of breaking my friend Bernie's personal best time of 2:45:24. During my long training runs, on the advice of Bernie himself, I drank Gatorade, which provides 14 g of precious carbohydrate energy per 8-ounce serving. I learned to appreciate just how much that sports drink helped me when I ran out of it during a 20-mile training run and bonked so badly that I had to stop at a gas station and call my girlfriend to beg a ride home.

Despite the setback I took comfort in knowing that I couldn't run out of sports drink in the race itself because there would be well-stocked aid stations positioned at every mile or so. I neglected, however, to find out exactly which sports drink would be served at those aid stations and to plan my race fueling strategy accordingly. I just took what was offered, which turned out to be Ultima Replenisher, a low-calorie sports drink that provides only 2.5 g of carbs per 8 ounces. Deprived of four-fifths of the energy they were accustomed to receiving while I ran, my muscles panicked and slowly shut down.

1

By the midpoint of the race I already knew I was in trouble. At 19 miles I was walking. Disgusted with myself, I tore off my race number, abandoned the course, and, with a feeling of déjà vu, called my brother Sean's cell phone (my girlfriend hadn't made the trip) from a pay phone outside a supermarket. Sean was waiting for me at the finish line, but I was going to tell him to come fetch me. No answer. I then realized that the only way to escape my nightmare was to finish the race, so I did, somehow, a scant 53 *minutes* off my goal time.

This was my rude welcome to what I like to call the Wall-Hitters Club. It is not an exclusive club. In fact, three out of four participants in any given marathon slow down significantly in the second half of the race, or "hit the wall." Hitting the wall in half marathons is less common but still far more common than in shorter events. Most often runners hit the wall after mile 20 in marathons and after mile 10 in half marathons, but some hit it sooner, as I did in my maiden 26.2-miler. The wall does not discriminate by talent or experience level or by any other factor. Runners are almost as likely to hit the wall in their tenth marathon or half marathon as they are in their first. Runners at the front of the race are as likely to hit the wall as runners at the back. Men and women of all ages are equally vulnerable. Maybe you've got your own story or you're hoping to avoid the wall in your first race; either way, this book will help you.

Like most runners who experience disastrous first marathons, I did not give up but instead climbed back on the horse and tried again. And again. Learning from past mistakes I was eventually able to figure out how to get beyond the wall and I've since run many satisfying marathons. I also became a professional running coach so I could help other runners break through the wall. Along the way I developed a special interest in the nutritional aspect of overcoming the wall and got myself certified as a sports nutritionist as well. I've since served as a consultant to several sports nutrition companies, authored a few books on endurance nutrition, including *Performance Nutrition for Runners* and *Racing Weight*, and provided nutritional advice to world-class runners, including Kara Goucher and Ryan Hall.

There are three main causes of hitting the wall. One is lack of fitness. Naturally, if you don't train properly for a marathon or half marathon your chances of running out of gas before you finish are greater. A second cause of hitting the wall is poor pacing. Marathons and half marathons are long enough that it's difficult for even experienced runners to accurately judge the most aggressive pace they can sustain from start to finish. Misjudging by as little as 1 percent and starting a marathon or half marathon just 5 seconds per mile too fast could bring on a catastrophe of fatigue with a few miles to go.

A third major cause of hitting the wall is a very broad category that we might file under the heading "Nutritional Errors." These are not limited to in-race mistakes such as taking in too little, too much, or the wrong types of fluid and fuel but also encompass training mistakes such as failing to consume proper recovery nutrition after hard workouts. My experience as an athlete, coach, and sports nutritionist has taught me that nutrition-related missteps are the most common cause of repeated encounters with the wall. They are also the most *overlooked* cause of disappointing marathons and half marathons (runners often never realize what they've done wrong) and are therefore in many instances the trickiest to solve as well. And it's not just nutrition-related mistakes per se that land runners in trouble but also nutrition-related missed opportunities stemming from lack of knowledge. (For example, did you know that relying on sports drinks too heavily in workouts could limit your body's fitness-building adaptations to training?)

The solution to bad pacing is relatively straightforward. If you ran too aggressively in your last race, try running more conservatively in your next one. Training properly so that you carry enough fitness into longer races to escape the wall is also something less than rocket science. There are lots of good books on marathon and half-marathon training. But a focused and comprehensive source of up-to-date information on fueling for these longer running events has been lacking. Long aware of this unfortunate gap, I have made it my mission to supply such a resource, which is now in your hands.

MARATHONS AND HALF MARATHONS are more popular than ever. Runners are attracted to these events because they represent the sport's ultimate challenge. Shorter races such as 5Ks and 10Ks are challenging in their own ways, but they are not as challenging as longer races because there is no wall.

The challenge of marathons and half marathons is fundamentally metabolic in nature. To hit the wall is to run out of energy, which, of course, comes from food. The marathon especially tests the human body's capacity to store, economize, and utilize fuel derived from food. A runner can hit the wall in a race of any distance if he or she paces it poorly. I've seen runners hit the wall in 400-meter sprints. But hitting the wall is rare in races of up to 10K in distance because these events do not test the limits of human metabolism. With sensible pacing there is little risk of blowing up in such races.

Most runners recognize that longer races are a largely nutritional challenge. Fewer, however, understand that success in marathons and half marathons depends as much on what one eats while preparing for such events as it does on what one drinks during them. For every runner who hits the wall because of his or her failure to consume enough carbohydrate during the race, there are several who hit the wall because of their failure to consume enough carbs in their everyday training diet. To truly minimize your chances of hitting the wall in your next marathon or half marathon you need to choose the right things to put into your body before, during, and after every training run; at different points along the training process; during the critical last two weeks before an event; during the even more critical final twenty-four hours; and within the race itself.

As a marathon and/or half-marathon runner you should put as much thought and discipline into your diet and fueling practices as you put into your training, but chances are you don't—yet. That's nothing to be ashamed of, for you are not alone. This is precisely why so many bad marathons and half marathons are to be blamed on nutritional mistakes and missed opportunities.

There are two reasons for the failure of runners to take nutrition as seriously as they take their training. The first relates to why we run, and that's because we love running and are highly motivated to train hard in pursuit of challenging race goals. Training hard comes relatively easily to us. But the motivation and the discipline that are required to train hard and the motivation and the discipline that are required to eat carefully are two different animals. As a rule, we runners have far more motivation and discipline for exercise than the general population does, but we do not have more motivation and discipline for eating carefully. And we all know that the average person's level of motivation and discipline to eat carefully is not especially high!

The second reason many of us runners don't take nutrition as seriously as we take our training is that we aren't *really* convinced that nutrition is equally important. We may give lip service to the idea, but we don't embrace it in our heart. This is understandable. After all, there are many successful runners who train hard and have a poor diet, but there aren't any successful runners who have a terrific diet and don't train hard. Training *is* more important than diet in the sense that, if you're only going to do one thing right—train or eat—you are better off training right. But if your desire is to be the best runner you can be, then nutrition really is just as important as training, because you can't run the best marathon or half marathon you're capable of without nailing it. The large and ever-growing membership of the Wall-Hitters Club proves it.

As a sports nutritionist and nutrition writer I spend a lot of time talking to and educating runners about nutrition. In doing so I am repeatedly struck by how much help the majority of runners need in this area. There's so much that even many experienced and highly competitive runners don't know. (I can recall being the first person to inform a particular Olympic runner that taking in caffeine before a race wouldn't help her performance unless she had ingested zero caffeine for at least a week beforehand.) And today the problem is worse than ever, because over the past decade there have been many important advances in nutritional best practices for marathon and half-marathon training and competition—advances that have achieved little penetration in the general distance-running population. A runner whose nutrition regimen was "state of the art" in 2002 but hasn't changed since then is not getting the benefit of a number of effective practices that have come along in the meantime.

It's not entirely the fault of runners themselves that marathon and half-marathon nutrition practices generally lag behind training practices (although, as you'll see in Chapter 9, I believe most runners could train more effectively too). It's also the fault of sports nutritionists like me. If nourishing and fueling the body properly is difficult, then my fellow professionals and I haven't done enough to make it easier. Runners understand plans and programs. Give a runner a good training plan and he or she will do the rest. In order to be practiced effectively, the "new rules" of marathon and half-marathon nutrition must be presented to runners in the simplest, most programmatic way possible. The purpose of this book is to do just that for you.

While many runners like to be told exactly how to train for their races, few runners want to be told exactly what to eat and drink throughout the process of training for and completing a marathon or half marathon. That's not even possible given the variety of tastes and dietary restrictions and lifestyles in the running population. But what is possible is the provision of simple, concrete nutritional guidelines that runners can use to make the fueling dimension of the marathon and half marathon experience nearly as systematic as the training and race execution dimensions. This book is intended to be the closest thing possible to a complete nutrition plan for these events.

Actually, it's a little more than that. Training and nutrition are not only coequal in their influence on race outcomes but they also influence each other. So what every runner really needs is an integrated training and nutrition plan for marathons and half marathons. This book, which is divided into three parts, culminates in the presentation of a selection of such plans in the final chapters. The preceding chapters will take you step by step toward that destination.

Part One addresses the two most important nutritional objectives of marathon and half-marathon training: consuming enough carbohydrate to get the most out of your training and maintaining the high level of overall diet quality needed to shed excess body fat and get down to your optimal racing weight. Together, these two key features of the proper diet for marathon or half-marathon training—high carbohydrate intake and high diet quality—comprise what I call the Two-Rule Diet. In Chapter 3 I will show you how to implement the Two-Rule Diet by recommending specific meals and snacks that are consistent with it. These are the nutritional equivalents of key workouts.

Part Two covers the umbrella topic of performance nutrition, which encompasses the critical matters of nutrition before, during, and after workouts; nutrition during the one- to three-week "taper" period before a race; immediate pre-race nutrition; fueling during events; and postrace nutrition.

Finally, in Part Three I will address the training component of what I call nutrition-training synergy and show you how to train in the way that best complements your nutritional efforts to push back the wall. This part also presents three complete integrated nutrition and training plans for the half marathon and three more for the marathon.

In the following pages I'm going to expose you to many ideas that are unfamiliar to you, challenge some of the ideas about nutrition that are familiar to you, and ask you to do some things you have never done before. To accept what I am offering you will need to put some trust in me. How can you trust that the ideas I present are true and that the things I tell you to do will work? Because a great many runners have already used these ideas and methods successfully to tear down the wall and lift their running to the next level—some with my direct help, others by finding the same answers elsewhere. You will encounter a number of their stories in the pages to come. Now it's your turn.

PART ONE

THE
TWO-RULE
DIET

MEETING YOUR CARBOHYDRATE NEEDS

Ben Rapoport hit the wall during the 2005 New York City Marathon. It happened in the Bronx, around mile 17. The first half of the race had gone well. An experienced runner, Ben had passed the 13.1-mile mark in 1:31, on pace to qualify for Boston. But just a few miles down the road, the wheels came off. Ben's legs became leaden. The pain in his thighs was searing. He tried as hard as he could to maintain his pace, but it was impossible. He wound up running the second half of the race twenty minutes slower than the first and failing to punch his ticket to Boston.

Thousands of other participants in the New York City Marathon also hit the wall that day. But Ben Rapoport was different. He happened to be a brilliant twenty-five-year-old scientist in his second year of a joint program at Harvard Medical School and MIT, studying toward an MD and a PhD in electrical engineering. After his disappointing marathon experience Ben decided to channel his considerable brain power into figuring out how to avoid ever hitting the wall again. Five years later he published a scientific paper describing a calculator that he had invented to make hitting the wall avoidable not just for himself but for any runner.

11

To use the Rapoport Calculator, as it is known, a runner is first required to enter some basic information including his or her current body weight and VO2 max (a measure of aerobic fitness). The calculator uses this information to spit out three specific recommendations to avoid hitting the wall: an appropriate target pace for the marathon, an amount of extra carbohydrate to consume in the final days before the marathon, and an amount of carbohydrate to consume during the marathon.

All three of these recommendations share a common purpose, which is to ensure that the runner does not use up all of the glycogen—a metabolic fuel derived from dietary carbohydrate—in his or her muscles and liver before reaching the finish line. The recommended pace is that which the calculator predicts to be the fastest pace the runner can sustain without depleting his or her glycogen supplies in less than 26.2 miles, based on his or her fitness level. The prerace and in-race carbohydrate intake targets are intended to make adequate glycogen available for the marathon given the runner's size, recommended pace, and fitness level.

There are still some bugs left to be worked out of the Rapoport Calculator. When I used it I was told I could run a 2:12 marathon. Trust me: I can't. But while no simple formula can be counted on to get you beyond the wall, Ben Rapoport's calculator does offer a useful implicit definition of the wall: glycogen depletion. And defining a problem is always the first step toward overcoming it.

Glycogen stored in the muscles and liver is one of two forms in which carbohydrate exists in the body. The other form is glucose, which comes to the muscles from the bloodstream and is continuously replenished from liver glycogen stores. Carbohydrate—in both forms, glycogen and glucose—is one of two major energy sources for running. The second source of energy for running is fat, which is stored in the muscles along with glycogen and is also made available to the muscles through the bloodstream from adipose tissue.

The body stores enough carbohydrate to fuel 15 to 26 miles of running, but it stores enough fat to fuel more than 100 miles of running. So together the body's fat and carbohydrate resources are able to supply enough energy to fuel at least four and a half marathons. But if this true, why do runners routinely hit the wall before they get to the finish line?

The problem is that runners do not have to deplete *both* their fat *and* their carbohydrate stores to hit the wall. Running low on carbohydrate fuel alone will do the job. In particular, running low on glycogen in the active muscles will accomplish this, since the body normally balances glycogen and glucose use during exercise to ensure that glycogen runs low first. What's more, the active muscles cannot work around the problem of limited carbohydrate stores by choosing to rely on fat to conserve carbs. Fuel source selection in the muscles is determined through automatic mechanisms that are governed primarily by running intensity. The faster you run, the more your muscles rely on carbohydrate. All runners burn some carbs when running at their marathon or half-marathon pace, so the longer you continue running at this pace, the more the glycogen stores in your working muscles are diminished. If the available glycogen stores fall too low before you finish, the active muscles send signals to the brain that trigger fatigue.

Worse, the muscles and liver do not have to run out of glycogen completely for exhaustion to occur. In fact, total glycogen depletion never happens. If it did, the runner's whole body would seize up in a terrible cramp known as muscle rigor. The reason you've never seen or experienced muscle rigor is that the body has a built-in protective mechanism to prevent it from happening. As I've hinted, this mechanism involves the transmission of chemical signals from the muscles to the brain that cause the runner to experience a perception of fatigue when glycogen stores are low but not yet fully depleted. Low glycogen is not the only factor that stimulates fatigue perceptions, but it is believed to be responsible for most episodes of hitting the wall in longer races. Other factors include muscle damage, core body temperature increase, and even fatigue within the brain itself.

Glycogen availability is the greatest metabolic limiter to marathon performance. To finish a marathon without hitting the wall you need to be able to sustain your goal pace without running too low on glycogen. As we've seen, this is an objective that marathon runners fail to achieve in approximately three out of every four cases. Both hitting the wall and glycogen depletion as a specific cause of hitting the wall are less common in half marathons than full marathons but are hardly unusual at the 13.1-mile distance.

Training methods and nutritional practices can delay glycogen depletion in marathons and half marathons in a variety of ways. In Chapter 10 we will discuss the training side of the solution. But our primary interest in this book is the nutritional side of solving the wall.

On the nutrition side, there are two rules governing everyday diet that will help you avoid glycogen depletion in races. Together these two rules comprise what I call the Two-Rule Diet for runners. In the present chapter we will discuss the first of these rules, which is getting the right amount of carbohydrate energy in your everyday diet to fully power the training process. A diet that supplies sufficient carbohydrate enhances training in much the same way that consumption of supplemental carbs in a sports drink or energy gels enhances race performance. In a race, taking in supplemental carbs provides an extra energy source that allows you to run faster and farther before you run out of fuel. Similarly, in training, eating enough carbohydrate every day will allow you to train harder, better absorb the stress of your training, and perform better in important workouts than you would without adequate carbohydrate intake.

AN ENERGY CRISIS

Simply put, carbohydrate is the most important energy source, or macronutrient, for runners who are training for marathons and half marathons. This fact has been known for more than a century, but lately it has been obscured by the ripple effects of a general decline in carbohydrate's reputation. Many runners today do not consume the right amount of carbohydrate to support their training. Some of these runners have not been taught how important carbohydrate is and how much of it they need. Others consciously limit their carbohydrate intake because they have been misled to believe that carbs are bad. To appreciate how this unfortunate situation came about it's helpful to review a little nutritional history.

In 1924 a team of researchers from Harvard University took blood samples from runners at the finish line of the Boston Marathon and found that those runners showing the most extreme signs of exhaustion invariably had blood glucose levels low enough to be classified as hypoglycemic. By this time it had already been shown by other scientists that endurance athletes (that is, cyclists, runners, and swimmers who compete in races lasting longer than a couple of minutes) performed significantly better in fitness tests after maintaining a high-carb diet than after maintaining a high-fat diet. The next year the same team of Harvard researchers encouraged some runners to train on high-carbohydrate diets in preparation for the 1925 Boston Marathon and also supplied some participants with sugar candies. Blood samples taken at the finish line this time revealed that runners hopped up on extra carbs had higher blood glucose levels than did those who had not trained on high-carb diets or eaten sugar candies during the race.

Subsequently a pair of Danish researchers, Erik Christensen and Ole Hansen, took the next step and actually quantified the effects of carbohydrate on endurance performance. They placed volunteers on either a low-carb, moderate-carb, or high-carb diet for one week, at the end of which all of the subjects were required to pedal a stationary bicycle to exhaustion at a fixed high intensity. On average the subjects lasted for just 81 minutes after a week of low-carb eating, compared to 206 minutes after seven days of carbohydrate feasting.

The reason for these effects remained a mystery for almost thirty years, until a group of Swedish researchers led by Jonas Bergstrom discovered that glycogen was the crucial link. In a landmark study, Bergstrom depleted the muscle glycogen stores of subjects with exhaustive exercise. As in the earlier study by Christensen and Hansen, the subjects were then placed on either a low-carb, moderate-carb, or high-carb diet and subjected to a stationary bike ride to exhaustion at a fixed intensity. The difference was that this time measurements of glycogen concentration were taken in each subject's quadriceps muscles. The average times to exhaustion in the low-carb, moderate-carb, and high-carb groups were 59 minutes, 126 minutes, and 189 minutes respectively, and there was a significant correlation between initial muscle glycogen concentrations and time to exhaustion.

Bergstrom had shown that maximizing muscle glycogen stores was a key to pushing back the wall of fatigue in endurance exercise, and that a high level of carbohydrate intake was a key to maximizing muscle glycogen stores. After the publication of this study in 1967, high-carbohydrate diets became widely used by serious endurance athletes around the world. In 1972 Frank Shorter practiced "carbohydrate loading" before winning the Olympic Marathon in Munich and the method was subsequently emulated by American runners of all ability and experience levels.

CARBOHYDRATE ATTACKED AND DEFENDED

In the first several decades after their discovery, all three macronutrients—protein, carbohydrate, and fat—were considered "good." They were essential for life, after all, and the more scientists learned about their effects in the body, the more their benefits were appreciated. But research conducted in the 1950s established a link between dietary fat intake and the risk of developing heart disease. This linkage inspired nutrition authorities to generally advocate a low-fat diet, which was also a de facto high-carbohydrate diet. Suddenly fat was "bad."

Not everyone bought into the antifat doctrine, however. In the 1960s a New York City cardiologist named Robert Atkins stepped forward to defend fat and claim that carbohydrate was the true "bad" macronutrient, blaming sugars and starches in particular for America's rising rate of obesity. His 1972 book, *Dr. Atkins' Diet Revolution*, was a huge hit. Even so, the theory that fat makes us fat had the full weight (so to speak) of the medical establishment behind it, and low-fat diets remained far more popular than the low-carb Atkins plan.

In the late 1990s, however, Robert Atkins made a comeback. His low-carb eating plan and various spinoffs became the most popular weight-loss diet fad in history. One of those spinoffs, the Zone diet, which peddled an ideal macronutrient ratio of 40 percent carbohydrate, 30 percent fat, and 30 percent protein, even became popular among endurance athletes. For years the American College of Sports Medicine and other organs of the endurance sports nutrition establishment had recommended a macronutrient ratio of 60 percent carbohydrate, 20 percent protein, and 20 percent fat. Between 2001 and 2005 endurance sports publications and websites featured scores of articles defending the established high-carb doctrine against the Atkins and Zone threats. Leading sports nutritionists including Nancy Clark,

Monique Ryan, Ellen Coleman, and Kim Mueller warned athletes that while low-carb diets might be effective for weight loss in non-athletes, they were sure to sabotage the training of endurance athletes by chronically depressing their critical muscle glycogen stores. Most athletes seemed to listen.

No diet fad, no matter how successful, lasts forever. By 2005 Robert Atkins had died (reportedly weighing 260 pounds at the time of his passing), *Dr. Atkins' New Diet Revolution* had fallen off best-seller lists, Atkins Nutritionals, Inc. had filed for bankruptcy, and restaurants had gone back to wrapping their hamburgers in buns instead of lettuce leaves. Nevertheless, in the succeeding years it has become increasingly apparent that Robert Atkins succeeded in causing a permanent change in public perceptions of carbohydrate. Despite being the most abundant energy source in plant foods, carbohydrate retains mostly negative associations in the mind of the typical health-conscious eater today. In the realm of sports nutrition, an older generation of experts educated under the influence of the "Swedish school" has lost sway and been usurped to some degree by a new generation of gurus that came of age during Atkins's reign and continues to advocate Zone-like diets for runners and other endurance athletes.

Today's advocates of low-carbohydrate diets for runners believe that increasing the muscles' capacity to burn fat is the single most important objective of a runner's training and diet, and that a low-carb (or high-fat) diet is the diet that increases the muscles' fat-burning capacity most effectively. There is no question that the ability to burn fat at high rates during running has a positive effect on marathon and half-marathon performance. For example, a 2005 study conducted by researchers at Cal State University at Sacramento found a strong correlation between the capacity to sustain high rates of fat oxidation at faster speeds and personal best marathon times in a group of twelve runners. Other studies have demonstrated that training increases fat-burning capacity. Some evidence suggests that the maximum rate of fat burning is more than twice as high in well-trained runners as in nonrunners.

There is also no question that a high-fat diet increases fat-burning during running in men and women of all fitness levels. Research has consistently shown that when athletes increase their habitual fat intake, their muscles use more fat and less carbohydrate to meet their energy needs at low and moderate exercise intensities. Theoretically, these adaptations to a high-fat diet could increase endurance—or push back the wall—by sparing muscle glycogen and delaying glycogen depletion.

The effects of a high-fat diet on performance in long-distance running races have not been well studied. I speculate that using a high-fat, low-carb diet to increase fat reliance during running is likely to be of significant benefit to those who compete in ultra-endurance races (50 km runs and longer). At the marathon and half-marathon distances, such a diet may help some runners slightly while making no difference at all for others. Even this limited potential to boost performance might be enough to justify using a high-fat, low-carb diet if there was no downside to doing so—but there is a downside.

The problem is that, while a high-fat diet may slightly increase endurance in a single prolonged bout of running, it reduces everyday training capacity. For you this means that the same training regimen that makes you feel strong and energized on a high-carbohydrate diet will wear you down on a high-fat diet. Runners on low-carb, high-fat diets lose more from reduced training capacity than they gain from increased fat-burning capacity. For this reason I recommend that runners train on a high-carbohydrate diet and rely on a high-fat diet only during a brief period within the prerace "taper" phase, which is the topic of Chapter 5.

In 2004 researchers at the University of Birmingham, England, compared the effects of a moderate-carbohydrate diet (5.4 g of carbs daily, or 41 percent of total calories) and a high-carbohydrate diet (8.5 g daily, or 65 percent of total calories) on performance capacity during eleven days of intensified training in a group of runners. They found that intensified training worsened performance in a 16 km time trial after eleven days of moderate-carb eating, whereas performance was fully maintained on a high-carb diet.

Of course, no runner in his or her right mind will make a habit of suddenly increasing his or her training load for eleven days and then running a 16 km time trial. Nevertheless, this study provides clear evidence that a higher level of carbohydrate intake is associated with a higher level of training tolerance.

Real-world examples of this principle are abundant. In 2005 Chip Henry made two big commitments simultaneously: He started training for his first marathon and he put himself on the Atkins diet. He lost weight quickly, but he also lost his energy. After several weeks on his new diet and training regimens, Chip had a hard time getting out of bed in the morning, let alone running. Suspecting that his diet was to blame, Chip purchased a copy of *Chris Carmichael's Food for Fitness* and followed the author's high-carb eating recommendations. Within days Chip's split times for 400 m (one-lap) intervals at the track had dropped by ten seconds. He went on to finish the Las Vegas Marathon in 4:22. Chip continues to run marathons and half marathons today and continues to follow a high-carb diet.

Chip Henry's story is typical of what happens to runners when they go in for branded low-carb regimens such as the Atkins or the Zone diet. In 2002 researchers at Kingston University in England studied the effects of switching to the Zone diet on high-intensity running endurance in a group of young men. Before the switch, the men were able to run at 80 percent of VO2 max for 37:41 before quitting in exhaustion. After a week on the Zone diet, that time had dropped all the way down to 34:06—a 9.5 percent decline in high-intensity running endurance.

Despite all of the scientific and real-world evidence that runners can train more effectively on high-carb diets, there are many runners who follow the Paleo diet (which forbids the consumption of grains), the Zone diet, and other low-carb diets without any apparent negative effect on their training. There are many possible explanations for these cases. Some runners eat more carbohydrate than they think they do. Others don't train hard enough for carbohydrate restriction to hamper their training. Still others may be hindered without out realizing it.

This last possibility was demonstrated in a 2011 study that was conducted by researchers at Australia's Charles Sturt University. Ten healthy male volunteers participated in a two-day intervention. On day one the subjects performed a long workout designed to deplete their muscle glycogen stores. That same evening, they were fed either a high-carbohydrate meal to replenish their muscle glycogen stores or a low-carbohydrate meal to keep those stores low. The subjects were not aware that their meals were being manipulated in this fashion.

The following day the subjects completed another workout. This one was a sixty-minute run that included a 15 m sprint every minute. The subjects who had been fed a low-carbohydrate meal unknowingly started this workout with almost 47 percent less glycogen in their muscles than did those who had been fed the high-carb meal. They also covered 4.9 percent less total distance in the sixty-minute run and 8.1 percent less distance in the sprint segments of the workout.

In addition to measuring performance, the scientists overseeing the study took ratings of perceived exertion (or how hard the run felt) from the subjects as they performed the workout. Interestingly, those ratings were the same between the two groups. Even though they were getting their butts kicked, the glycogen-depleted subjects felt that the workout was no harder for them than the glycogen-replenished subjects felt it was for themselves. In other words, the glycogen-depleted subjects had no idea their performance was being compromised by their diet. This might be what's going on with many runners on relatively low-carb diets who report being satisfied with those diets. Chronically low muscle glycogen stores are sabotaging their performance and they don't even know it.

HIGH-CARB DIETS IN THE REAL WORLD

You should not base your training or nutritional practices solely on the results of scientific research. It's also important to consider the results of various practices in the real world. Most of the world's best runners use high-carb diets. As a group, the best runners the world has ever seen come from the Kalenjin tribe of Kenya. The typical Kenyan diet is extremely rich in carbohydrate. In 2004 scientists at Kenyatta University of Nairobi, Kenya analyzed the diets of a group of elite Kenyan runners during a week of intense training. The researchers found that more than 76 percent of the athletes' daily calories came from carbohydrate. Compare that to the typical American diet, which is less than 50 percent carbohydrate.

The staples of the Kenyan diet are cooked greens and other vegetables, fruit, tea with lots of milk, roasted goat and beef, and *ugali*, which is a thick cornmeal porridge that most East Africans eat daily. Fast food, fried snack chips, soft drinks, and candy are not staples of the Kenyan diet as they are of the American.

Breakfast is usually eaten after the first run of the day and is relatively light, consisting of fruit, buttered bread, and perhaps a couple of boiled eggs. Copious amounts of tea with whole milk are consumed with this meal and all Kenyan meals. It is an ideal postexercise recovery beverage, providing fluid and minerals for rehydration, carbohydrates to replenish glycogen stores, proteins for muscle tissue repair, some fat to replenish muscle triglyceride stores, and antioxidants to limit delayed-onset muscle soreness caused by free radicals.

Lunch is also relatively light, because it is eaten before the day's second training session. A typical menu is rice or boiled potatoes with cooked vegetables and a small portion of meat, again washed down with a large volume of tea and milk. As a whole, it's a veritable carbohydrate bomb.

If snacks are needed to keep hunger at bay until dinnertime, those snacks almost invariably consist of fruit—and yet more tea. Dinner is the big meal of the day. At its center is a generous helping of *ugali*, which provides a whopping 22 g of carbohydrate per ounce. This is usually topped with a stew containing a lot of vegetables and a little meat. And to drink? Tea, of course.

It is fortunate for Kenyan runners that the traditional Kenyan diet they are brought up on is also the ideal running diet. They don't have to discover the benefits of high-carb eating the hard way, as many Western runners do. The silver lining for Western runners is that they get to enjoy the breakthrough that comes with a switch to a high-carb diet.

Mark Percy experienced such a breakthrough when he was training for the New York City Marathon in 2000. Mark's wife, Kate, was schooled in French cooking. She prepared lots of dinners centered on meat dishes with heavy sauces, which her husband greatly enjoyed but which did not supply the amount of carbohydrate that was needed to support his training. When Mark was halfway through the process of preparing for his race his fitness stagnated and he began to feel tired all the time, not just in his runs but throughout the day as well. Concerned, Kate did some reading on sports nutrition and identified the problem. She overhauled Mark's diet, adding carb-rich foods such as basmati rice, couscous, quinoa, sweet potatoes, and pasta to the dinners she made and also encouraging him to start each day with a carb-rich meal such as oatmeal porridge.

Things turned around for Mark almost immediately. His workouts improved, his energy returned, and he began to enjoy his training once again. When race day came around he improved his personal best marathon time by twenty minutes. Kate went on to become a sports dietitian and authored a book, titled *Go Faster Food*.

YOUR CARBOHYDRATE TARGET

My intent in describing the diet of Kenya's great Kalenjin runners is not to present it as an ideal for all runners to follow. I offer it as another piece of evidence that a high-carbohydrate diet is generally the right way to go for runners training for marathons or half marathons. There is no better possible validation for the research finding that a high-carb diet increases training capacity than the fact that the world's best runners get more than three-fourths of their daily calories from carbs. This does not mean, however, that every runner should maintain a 76 percent carb diet. Exactly how much carbohydrate should you aim to consume daily?

For the same reason that runners generally need more carbohydrate than nonathletes, runners with very heavy training loads need more carbohydrate than runners with more moderate training loads. The more you train, the more carbs your body uses, and the more carbohydrate your body uses, the more carbs you need to eat to maintain adequate muscle glycogen stores.

Few runners need as much carbohydrate as do the Kalenjins, whose diet was analyzed in the Kenyatta University study. These athletes consumed more than 10 g of carbohydrate per kilogram of body weight each day. Interestingly, runners from the only nation that rivals Kenya in running success, Ethiopia, eat similar amounts of carbohydrate. Other research has shown that 10 g/kg is the largest amount of carbohydrate that a trained runner is able to benefit from. Such a large amount of carbohydrate is only ever needed to elevate muscle glycogen stores to the maximum possible level during a brief prerace "carbo loading" period that follows a sharp reduction in training from peak workloads. When 10 g/kg of carbs are consumed in any other circumstances, the excess that cannot be stored as glycogen is converted to fat and stored in adipose tissue. Any runner who tried to consume more carbs would also find it very difficult, if not impossible, to meet the body's fat and protein requirements without gaining weight, or to maintain a steady weight without failing to meet the body's fat or protein requirements. Indeed, the Kalenjin runners who were studied got only 10 percent of their calories from protein, barely meeting the World Health Organization's minimum standard for health.

The maximum amount of carbohydrate that runners require to maintain performance during normal training is approximately 8 g/kg per day, and only the hardest-training runners need this much. One of the world's leading authorities on the macronutrient needs of endurance athletes, the Australian Institute of Sport's Louise Burke, has established 5 g/kg per day as a sensible target for athletes with moderate training loads. Runners who train very lightly (for example, running 20 miles per week and doing no cross-training) may be able to get by on as little as 3 g/kg. For such runners, a target of 4 g/kg would offer extra insurance against inadequacy without any downside, again provided that those carbs came mostly from veggies, fruits, and whole grains.

Table 1.1 presents recommended daily carbohydrate intake targets for runners with different training loads. The relatively broad ranges reflect the fact that science has not so far come up with any strict formula for carbohydrate intake. In fact, the available science suggests that most runners can train equally well at a range of carbohydrate intake levels, as long as they meet a certain minimum for their body weight and training volume.

Let's see what these recommendations look like for a hypothetical runner. Suppose this runner—let's call him John—weighs 165 pounds (75 kg) and is currently running about forty-five minutes a day in

TABLE 1.1 *RECOMMENDED CARBOHYDRATE INTAKE*

AVERAGE DAILY TRAINING TIME (RUNNING AND OTHER ACTIVITIES)	DAILY CARBOHYDRATE TARGET
30–45 minutes	3–4 g/kg
46–60 minutes	4–5 g/kg
61–75 minutes	5–6 g/kg
76–90 minutes	6–7 g/kg
90–120 minutes	7–8 g/kg
>120 minutes	8–10 g/kg

training for a half marathon. According to the guidelines in Table 4.1, John should aim to consume 4 to 5 g of carbohydrate per kilogram of body weight each day. Because John is at the low end of the training volume range associated with this carbohydrate intake range, 4 g/kg daily should be plenty. Multiplying this figure by John's weight, we get a recommended daily carbohydrate intake of 300 g. Because each gram of carbohydrate supplies 4 calories, this value equates to 1,200 carbohydrate calories per day.

What does it take to get 300 g of carbohydrate? Here's one example of a day's eating menu that meets this requirement: a cup of old-fashioned oatmeal with sliced banana and an 8-ounce glass of orange juice for breakfast; a small tub of strawberry yogurt as a postrun recovery snack; a bowl of tomato soup and a slice of toasted whole wheat bread with hummus for lunch; a handful of cashews as an afternoon snack; a chicken and broccoli stir-fry with one cup of brown rice for dinner; and an apple for dessert.

To maintain his or her body weight, a 165-pound runner who trains forty-five minutes per day must consume approximately 2,650 calories per day. So this runner needs to get about 45 percent of his daily calories from carbs. I've provided these numbers for the sake of illustration. You do not need to calculate your total daily calorie needs to determine how much carbohydrate to include in your diet. You need only know your weight and how much running (and other exercise) you typically do.

These numbers happen to be very close to those that are provided by the typical American diet, which, as mentioned, is roughly 50 percent carbohydrate and supplies roughly 4 g of carbohydrate per kilogram of body weight. Therefore, our hypothetical runner does not have to make any special effort to get enough carbohydrate. But runners who train more than sixty minutes per day on average cannot meet their carbohydrate needs of 5 g/kg per day or more on the typical American diet (unless they overeat). If you train at this level you will probably have to go a bit out of your way to get all the carbs you need. Of course, you shouldn't eat the typical American diet anyway. This diet's insufficient carbohydrate supply to hard-training runners is just one more reason to break away from it.

The diet quality guidelines for losing excess body fat that I will present in the next chapter (rule number two of the Two-Rule Diet) encourage a higher level of carbohydrate intake than is associated with the typical American diet. In Chapter 4 I will present sample meal plans that will enable you to meet your carbohydrate needs and the diet quality requirements for body fat loss simultaneously.

WHAT ABOUT FAT AND PROTEIN?

Although carbohydrate is the most important macronutrient for runners training for marathons and half marathons, minimum levels of fat and protein are required for optimal training as well. These standards are more easily met.

Running increases protein needs above the levels needed by sedentary individuals in two ways. First, protein supplies about 5 percent of the energy the muscles use during running. Second, running damages muscle proteins, which must then be replaced during the post-workout recovery period. The sum effect of these processes on protein needs, however, is small. There is broad agreement among experts on protein metabolism that 1 g of protein per kilogram of body weight daily is sufficient for most endurance athletes, whereas 1.6 g/kg is the most needed by any endurance athlete. The average American adult takes in approximately 1.3 g of protein per kilogram of body weight daily. Contrary to popular belief, vegetarians and vegans get about the same amount of protein as omnivores, hence more than enough to support marathon or half-marathon training.

Minimum fat intake requirements are not well established for endurance athletes. The American College of Sports Medicine recommends that athletes get at least 20 percent of their daily calories from fat. Some research suggests that lower fat intake levels are associated with reduced performance and increased injury risk, at least in female runners, but this appears to be the case not because fat intake itself is inadequate but rather because total energy intake is too low.

More important than the total amount of fat in the diet is the amount of omega-3 fats, which are classified as essential nutrients because they are the only fats the body cannot manufacture for itself. Most Americans do not consume enough omega-3s, which are found in high concentrations in only a handful of foods, including salmon, halibut, tuna, almonds, walnuts, kale, and spinach. For this reason I recommend that all runners consume an omega-3 supplement such as fish oil or flaxseed oil daily. Studies have linked such supplements to reduced muscle tissue inflammation and oxidative stress after exercise. Don't think of these products as an excuse not to eat omega-3-rich real foods, however. No supplement ever truly substitutes for natural whole foods.

Theoretically, you could also meet your daily carbohydrate needs with a diet that's full of low-quality processed foods such as snack chips and low in natural, whole foods such as vegetables. Should you? Of course not. As I've suggested, meeting your carbohydrate needs so you can get the most out of your training is just one of two critical components of the proper everyday diet for marathon and half-marathon training. The second rule of my Two-Rule Diet for runners is to maximize your overall diet quality so you can shed excess body fat and get down to your optimal racing weight.

GETTING LEAN

CHAPTER 2

Dathan Ritzenhein was already an accomplished world-class runner when he decided to run his first marathon—the 2006 New York City Marathon. His résumé at the age of twenty-four included four national championship titles at the high school, college, and professional levels and an Olympic Games appearance. When he made the decision to move up to the marathon, "Ritz" had never raced farther than 12 km (7.4 miles), so he was concerned about fueling his body sufficiently to survive the 110-mile training weeks his coach had scheduled for him—and to avoid the wall on race day. *Too* concerned, as it turned out.

"I was so paranoid about running low on energy that I ate whatever I saw," Dathan recalled later on his blog.

Ritz started the race weighing 130 pounds, which doesn't sound very heavy but it was 10 pounds above his usual racing weight. He ran the first half at a steady five minutes per mile, hanging in the shadow of the race leaders. So far, so good. When eventual winner Marilson Gomes dos Santos surged a few miles later, Ritz was able to accelerate, too, covering the distance between the 25 km and 30 km marks in a blistering 14:53. Then he hit the wall. Feeling every ounce of the extra weight he carried, Dathan slogged through the distance between the 35 km and 40 km marks in 17:17, and slowed down even more in the final mile.

He learned his lesson. When Ritz returned to New York City the following year for the U.S. Olympic trials marathon he weighed 121 pounds, thanks to a cleaned-up diet. On a tougher course he ran three minutes faster than he had in his debut marathon, finishing second behind Ryan Hall and qualifying for his second Olympics.

Body weight is the enemy of running performance. Running is, after all, a continuous fight against gravity. With every stride you take your body must be lifted completely off the ground, because all of the progress you make when running is made while your body is airborne. What's more, your body also must be accelerated forward with every stride because it loses momentum upon each foot landing. The energy cost of accelerating your body forward is proportional to how much you weigh. The same goes for the energy cost of lifting your body upward against gravity. So the heavier you are, the more fuel you burn when running at any given speed—and the more fuel you burn, the sooner you hit the wall.

A runner who weighs 160 pounds has to muster approximately 6.5 percent more energy to run the same pace as a runner weighing 150 pounds. No wonder the typical elite male marathon runner weighs only 125 pounds, while the typical elite female marathon runner tips the scales at just 110 pounds.

Studies involving elite runners have shown that the very best runners tend to be the leanest of the lean. For example, a 2009 study found that small differences in body fat percentage among two dozen elite runners from Ethiopia accounted for the lion's share of differences in their race times. All of these runners were very lean and very fast, but those with the least body fat were the fastest.

Most runners don't have the right genes to get as lean or light as the world's best runners. But chances are you can probably get a little leaner and lighter than you are today and get a little faster as a result. Indeed, because of the link between body weight and performance, losing excess weight should be one of the highest priorities of every runner seeking to run his or her best marathon or half marathon. A four-hour marathoner who loses 10 pounds without any change in fitness would run her next marathon in 3:45. That's too big an opportunity to pass up!

Even if you're already fairly lean you may benefit from a small amount of weight loss in the lead-up to your next race. That's because there is a difference between a person's *healthy body weight range* and a runner's *ideal racing weight*. A runner's ideal racing weight usually falls at the low end of what doctors consider to be the healthy body weight range for an individual of a given height. For example, according to the calculations used by the U.S. government, the healthy body weight range for a person who is six feet, one inch tall (which happens to be my height) is 140 to 188 pounds. I know from experience that my ideal racing weight is 154 pounds, which falls in the lower third of that range. I've never tried to run a marathon at 188 pounds and I hope I never have to!

A certain amount of body fat is needed for good health. You can have somewhat more than this minimum amount of essential fat on your body (as nearly everyone does) and still be very healthy. But your ideal racing weight is defined as your body weight when you are very close to having the minimum amount of body fat you need for good health. Any additional fat above that amount is just dead weight that slows you down, even if it doesn't make you less healthy.

THE COMPENSATION EFFECT

Both training and diet contribute toward the attainment of a runner's optimal racing weight during the process of preparing for a marathon or half marathon. As I will explain in Chapter 9, the right approach to training will burn excess fat off your body in addition to building fitness. But smart training alone won't reduce your weight to the optimal level for racing. To get all the way there you must eat right, too. In fact, runners generally have to eat more carefully to reach their optimal racing weight than must nonrunners to reach a "merely" healthy body weight. One of the reasons is, again, that a runner's optimal racing weight is in most cases significantly lower than the upper limit of his or her healthy body weight range. A second reason has to do with a phenomenon called the compensation effect.

The compensation effect is the tendency of individuals to eat more when they exercise more. Appetite is linked to activity level. Men and especially women often lose less weight than they expect to lose through increases in exercise because they become hungrier and eat more. Runners are not exempt from the compensation effect, which has been known to cause some runners to actually *gain* weight while training for a marathon or half marathon despite burning many more calories than they do at other times. To overcome the compensation effect and reach your optimal racing weight you may have to make even better dietary choices than you do at other times.

It's true that some runners with favorable genes (who are known as exercise responders) lose a little weight "automatically" as they increase their training in preparation for a marathon or half marathon, even if their diet leaves something to be desired. Too often these runners interpret any amount of training-induced weight loss as proof that they are doing enough to manage their weight for running performance and can get away with continuing to eat somewhat carelessly. Indeed, the competitive running culture has traditionally taken a certain amount of pride in the apparent power of high-mileage training to overcome any potential negative effects of unhealthy eating habits. In his classic 1978 novel *Once a Runner*, John L. Parker Jr. wrote, "If the furnace is hot enough, anything burns, even Big Macs." That phrase—"If the furnace is hot enough, anything burns"—has remained a slogan of junk-eating competitive runners ever since.

Those runners who are naturally lean and/or who maintain particularly high training loads are the ones who are most easily fooled into believing that they can eat a sloppy diet without suffering any consequences. After all, when they look in the mirror they don't *see* any extra fat on their body. Bill Rodgers famously filled his belly with gallons of mayonnaise, buckets of sugary breakfast cereals, chocolate chip cookies, snack chips, soft drinks, and gin and tonics. Rodgers's eight career victories in the Boston and the New York City marathons might seem to prove that his diet did not hurt him. But it's possible—even likely, I think—that with a better diet Bill Rodgers would have become even leaner than he was and run even faster than he did.

There are noteworthy examples of elite runners who had questionable eating habits before taking a leap of faith and cleaning up their diet. The results of these individual experiments suggest that no runner truly gets away with loose nutritional standards. One such case is that of Chris Solinsky, who despite eating a couple of frozen pizzas every week while running for the University of Wisconsin won five individual NCAA titles. With that kind of success Solinsky had as much reason as any runner to believe that his diet wasn't holding him back one bit. But at 165 pounds he was heavy for a runner of his caliber, and his consciousness of this fact perhaps made him a little more open to experimenting with stricter nutritional standards than 128-pound Bill Rodgers ever was. After turning professional and moving to Portland, Oregon, to run for Nike, Solinsky cut out the frozen pizzas, started cooking for himself more, and increased his fruit and vegetable intake. Sure enough, he lost a few pounds and took a quantum leap forward as a runner, setting an American record of 26:59 for 10,000 meters in 2010.

Chris Solinsky was running between 100 and 120 miles per week when he set his record. If a runner like him cannot reach his optimal racing weight without eating carefully, then no runner can. This hard reality is much more widely accepted among today's elite runners than it was among runners of Bill Rodgers's generation. Solinsky represents a new breed of runners who understand that any runner who takes his diet as seriously as he takes his training will be leaner and race better than a runner who considers hard training a license to eat whatever he wants. Whatever your goals, whether you're a lifelong runner like Solinsky or a weekend warrior, or you're training for a longer race for the first time, paying attention to your weight and running at your leanest will help you avoid hitting the wall.

There are right ways and wrong ways to pursue weight loss as a runner. The usual dieter's approach of sharply reducing overall food intake is the wrong way. The problem for runners is that this approach deprives the body of the fuel it needs for training and recovery. It also exacerbates the compensation effect. If training hard makes a runner hungry, then training hard and eating less makes a runner intolerably hungry. To shed excess body fat while training for a marathon or half marathon without underfueling your body and driving yourself crazy with hunger, you cannot eat less. Instead you must follow the example of today's world-class runners such as Chris Solinsky and simply eat *better*. In other words, you need to focus more on the *quality* than on the *quantity* of the foods you eat.

DIET QUALITY GOES UP, WEIGHT COMES DOWN

Some foods are known to promote weight gain. It's the obvious stuff we all know about: snack chips, candy, soft drinks—call these low-quality foods. Other foods are known to prevent weight gain. Again, no surprises here: fruits, vegetables, whole grains—call these high-quality foods. Here's something you may not be aware of: The main reason low-quality foods promote weight gain is that they are calorically dense. This means they pack a lot of calories in a small amount of space—without a lot of nutritional value.

CALORIE DENSITY

Appetite is regulated not only by the number of calories we eat but also by the volume of food we eat. Therefore we tend to eat more calories when we eat calorically dense foods. High-quality foods tend to prevent weight gain because their caloric density is low. They contain fewer calories than low-quality foods do in an equal amount of space, so they satisfy our appetite with fewer calories.

If you maintain a diet that consists primarily of high-quality foods and allow your appetite to determine how much you eat, you will get enough calories to meet your energy needs for training and recovery but not so many calories that your body is able to hold onto the excess fat stores that stand between your current weight and your optimal racing weight. We are accustomed to thinking of appetite as unreliable—especially when the compensation effect is at play. Experts tell us that if we permit ourselves to eat as much as our hunger asks for, we inevitably eat too much. But the biological mechanisms that regulate appetite are the products of millions of years of evolution and they actually work quite well provided we eat the natural, high-quality foods we are meant to eat. It's only when we stray into the domain of unnaturally calorie-dense low-quality foods that our appetite can no longer be trusted.

Scientists began to seriously explore how different foods affect appetite in the mid-1990s. At that time Susanna Holt, a biochemist at the University of Sydney, Australia, conducted a study in which she fed 240 calories' worth of thirty-eight foods to volunteers on an empty stomach. After consuming a given food, the volunteers rated their hunger level every fifteen minutes for two hours and then ate as much (or as little) of a standardized meal as they desired. Holt counted the number of calories the subjects ate in these meals and combined this data with their hunger ratings to create a "satiety index" score for each of the thirty-eight foods tested. Those foods that were associated with the lowest hunger ratings and the smallest meals eaten two hours later earned the highest satiety index scores.

In addition to ranking the thirty-eight foods she tested individually, Holt identified some general characteristics of foods that predicted high satiety index scores. The characteristic that had the greatest impact on satiety was caloric density, with the least calorie-dense foods yielding the most satiety. Boiled potatoes had the highest satiety index score of any food that Holt tested. It takes 10 ounces of boiled potatoes to supply 240 calories. The least satiating food in Holt's study was doughnuts. It takes just 2 ounces of doughnuts to supply 240 calories.

Potatoes are, of course, a natural food, whereas doughnuts are processed. Holt did not look at the relationship between naturalness and satiety, or between processing and satiety, but if she had she would have found that natural foods generally had higher satiety index scores than do processed foods. There are exceptions, though.

Peanuts, which of course grow in the ground, earned a lower satiety index score than did potato chips, which are processed through frying. Likewise, jelly beans achieved a satiety index score that was higher than that of yogurt, which humans have eaten for thousands of years.

Do these results tell us that people are better off eating potato chips and jelly beans than peanuts and yogurt? Of course not. The short-term effects of specific foods on satiety and subsequent eating may not always be perfect indicators of the long-term effects of the same foods on body weight. Common sense tells us that artificial foods such as potato chips and jelly beans are far more likely to make us fat than are natural foods such as yogurt. While laboratory studies like the one that Susanna Holt did are valuable, more valuable still are studies that look at the effects of specific foods on body weight in the real world. Real-world studies have shown that, satiety index scores notwithstanding, the natural foods we think of as high-quality foods tend to prevent weight gain, whereas the processed foods we think of as low-quality foods promote weight gain.

One such study was performed in 2010 by a team of researchers led by Frank Hu at the Harvard School of Public Health. This study found that people who included more fruits, vegetables, nuts, and yogurt in their diet tended to gain less weight over a twenty-year period. Those who consumed more potato chips, soft drinks, and meat tended to gain more weight.

These findings surprised no one. The average third-grader could tell you that you might want to lay off the chips, burgers, and soda, and eat more fruit, vegetables, nuts, and yogurt, if you want to lose weight. Many runners who lack any special nutrition expertise instinctively make such changes when they make a commitment to lose weight. Murat Akman, a Turkish runner in his fifties, is one example. Weighing 187 pounds and frustrated by recurring injuries resulting from running at that weight, Murat replaced all of the refined flour in his diet with whole-grain flour, gave up sweets and pastries, and also replaced fatty meats with leaner cuts. He lost 33 pounds in a few months and his injuries disappeared.

NUTRIENT DENSITY

A positive impact on body weight is not the only defining characteristic of high-quality foods. A second characteristic is *nutrient density*. A nutrient-dense food is one that contains large amounts of micronutrients that do not supply energy: vitamins, minerals, and antioxidants. It is possible that the high nutrient density of natural foods contributes to their beneficial effects on body weight. There is some evidence that certain micronutrients affect the brain's appetite control systems, and that micronutrient deficiencies increase appetite. This would explain why even those natural foods that are relatively calorie-dense or nonsatiating promote a lean body composition.

In any case, the vitamins, minerals, and antioxidants in natural foods provide many health benefits that go beyond their beneficial effect on body weight. An effort to rank foods by quality must therefore account for their nutrient density as well as their beneficial effect on body weight (which is generally associated with low calorie density). All natural foods are either low in calorie density or high in nutrient density or both, while most processed foods are just the opposite.

THE DIET QUALITY CONTINUUM

There are various ways to categorize foods. For the purpose of regulating diet quality I employ a classification system that arranges all of the world's foods into ten categories. These categories are, in order of decreasing quality:

1. Vegetables (including legumes)

2. Fruits

3. Nuts and seeds

4. Fish and lean meats

5. Whole grains

6. Dairy products

7. Refined grains

8. Fatty meats

9. Sweets

10. Fried foods

The first six foods on the continuum are high-quality foods, which means that all of them should be included in your diet, albeit in varying proportions, as I will discuss later in the chapter. The last four foods on the continuum are low-quality foods, some lower than others. As I suggested earlier, these rankings are determined by the calorie density, nutrient density, and naturalness of each food type. Let's take a closer look at each category of food before I discuss how to balance them to optimize your diet quality and attain your ideal racing weight.

HIGH-QUALITY FOODS

These six foods comprise the high-quality half of the diet quality continuum.

1. VEGETABLES

A vegetable is, by culinary tradition rather than scientific definition, an edible leaf (such as spinach), stem (such as broccoli), root (such as a potato), seed (such as a bean), or nonsweet fruit (such as a squash). You could live in splendid health if you ate nothing but vegetables. This cannot be said of any other category of food, and it is for this reason that I rank vegetables as the highest-quality food type.

Vegetables promote a lean body composition because they contain large amounts of fiber and water and are therefore highly satiating and not very calorie dense. They promote all-around health because they are rich in a wide variety of vitamins, minerals, and so-called phytonutrients, most of which function as antioxidants. There are several different types of vegetables and each type tends to be richer in certain nutrients and poorer in others. For example, beans are typically the most protein-rich vegetables, whereas green, leafy vegetables have the largest amounts of a number of micronutrients, including vitamin K and iron. In addition to eating a lot of vegetables generally it's a good idea to eat a wide *variety* of vegetables so you can benefit from the unique nutrient profile of each type.

No vegetable contains the essential vitamin B_{12}. Vegetables also are not the best sources of iron and a few other nutrients. For this reason it is best not to try to live on vegetables alone, although you should eat more vegetables than you do any other category of food.

2. FRUITS

Vegetables and fruits are often lumped together into a single category. And why not? They're very similar. Both are nutrient-rich plant foods that (with a few exceptions) can be eaten raw. Some veggies and fruits are indistinguishable. Tomatoes are fruits that are eaten like vegetables. Beets are vegetables whose sweet juice is consumed like fruit juices.

The nutritional makeup and health benefits of fruits and vegetables are very similar. Like vegetables and the nonsweet fruits that are considered vegetables, fruits have relatively low calorie densities and high satiety indices because of high fiber and water contents. They are also, like vegetables, packed with vitamins, minerals, and antioxidants. There are some differences, however. As a category, vegetables contain larger amounts of key minerals, including iron and calcium, whereas fruits as a category contain larger amounts of certain important vitamins, such as vitamin C.

Fruits generally contain less fat and protein and more carbohydrate than vegetables do. The carbs in vegetables and fruits also take different forms. Most of the carbs in vegetables are starches, whereas most of the carbs in fruits are sugars. While sugar has earned a bad name, the sugars in fruits are not bad. In fact, some epidemiological studies have found that fruit promotes a lean body composition even more effectively than do vegetables. Nevertheless, I rank vegetables one step higher than fruit in quality because there is slightly greater overall nutritional balance in vegetables as a category.

3. NUTS AND SEEDS

Nuts and seeds are among nature's most balanced energy sources, providing lots of healthy unsaturated fats, good amounts of protein, and some carbs as well. In combination, these macronutrients make nuts and seeds very energy dense, yet people who eat nuts and seeds regularly tend to be leaner than those who do not. Foods in this category are also nutrient dense, supplying an abundance of minerals such as magnesium, potassium, and zinc, along with B vitamins and other vitamins.

4. FISH AND LEAN MEATS

As I define it, this category includes all forms of wild-caught seafood; meat from grass-fed, organically produced, and/or free-range animals; eggs; and other meats that are less than 10 percent fat. I consider fish and lean meat to be high-quality foods because they are natural, nutrient dense, and only moderately calorie dense. Foods in this category are nature's best sources of protein and excellent sources of fat-soluble vitamins and minerals, including iron.

Fish and lean meat are controversial foods. Experts such as Colin Campbell, author of *The China Study*, contend that all animal foods are unhealthy and that optimal health is achievable only on a vegetarian diet. On the other side of the controversy are the likes of Loren Cordain, author of *The Paleo Diet*, who believes that because our Paleolithic ancestors ate lots of meat and seafood, we modern humans should, too.

My take on the subject is that consumption of fish and meat is clearly not necessary for optimal health or running performance. Research aside, the success of the many vegetarian and vegan runners in the world is proof of that. But the best scientific evidence suggests that wild fish and meats that are close in form to those that our ancestors consumed are in no way harmful to those who choose to eat them.

5. WHOLE GRAINS

Whole grains such as brown rice, whole wheat, corn, and oats comprise another category of foods that are not necessary in the human diet and that some runners and nonrunners choose to avoid without consequence. They are nevertheless high-quality foods whose consumption is associated with lower body weights and reduced risk of heart disease and diabetes. Whole grains are especially helpful to runners because they are nature's most concentrated sources of carbohydrate. Personally, I don't know how I would get all the carbs I need daily without them.

While whole grains are energy dense, they are also satiating because they contain lots of fiber and they promote stable blood glucose levels. Whole grains do not provide the abundance of phytonutrients that vegetables and fruits do, but they are good sources of many essential vitamins and minerals. Also, while most grains contain only small amounts of protein, they contain amino acids (protein building blocks) that are generally complementary to the amino acids in other plant foods (legumes especially). Thus a diet that includes both offers all the protein a person—even a runner—needs.

6. DAIRY PRODUCTS

Dairy products are calorie dense, high in fat, and only moderately satiating. Nevertheless, epidemiological studies have generally shown that regular consumption of dairy products is not associated with long-term weight gain. What's more, dairy consumption has consistently been shown to enhance fat loss and accelerate improvements in body composition in people following an energy-restricted weight-loss diet. It appears that the calcium in dairy products inhibits fat storage, while the abundance of high-quality protein promotes muscle retention. As I mentioned earlier, yogurt seems to be especially beneficial for body composition.

Dairy products are somewhat less natural than the food categories ranked higher on the diet quality continuum because they entered the human diet only a few thousand years ago. Most people who trace their ancestry to parts of the world where dairy consumption arrived even later cannot properly digest dairy products. Between 10 and 20 percent of American adults are lactose intolerant. Their body does not produce sufficient amounts of the enzyme that is needed to digest the lactose sugar in cow's milk. Because of this they suffer symptoms of gastrointestinal distress after consuming nonfermented dairy products. (Fermented dairy products such as yogurt are generally well tolerated by lactose-intolerant individuals because the lactase in them is essentially predigested.)

If you are comfortable eating and drinking dairy products, there is really no other reason not to include them in your diet, unless you're a vegan. Milk is nutrient dense, containing all twenty-two essential minerals and heavy concentrations of fat-soluble vitamins and B vitamins.

There is no clear difference in the health and body-composition effects of whole-milk dairy products and reduced-fat dairy products. If you are wary of the high saturated fat content of whole milk, you may consume reduced-fat alternatives with greater peace of mind, if not greater benefits. But be aware that some low-fat products, especially yogurts, can contain additional additives for texture or other qualities, to replace the fat. If you believe strongly in the principle of naturalness, you may choose whole-milk dairy products with greater satisfaction and no less benefit.

LOW-QUALITY FOODS

These four food categories comprise the low-quality half of the diet quality continuum.

7. REFINED GRAINS

A processed or refined grain is a grain that has been stripped of most of its non-energy nutrition. For example, white flour is made from wheat that has been stripped of its germ, removing most of the grain's natural fiber, vitamin, and mineral content and leaving behind its starch and a bit of protein. Refined grains such as white rice are much lower-quality foods than the natural whole grains they're made from and are less healthful. A study out of the Harvard School of Public Health found that men and women who ate more than two servings of brown rice (a whole grain) per week had a lower-than-average risk for type 2 diabetes, while those who ate five or more servings of white rice (a refined grain) per week had an above-average risk for the disease.

Minimizing your consumption of refined grains will help you maximize the improvements in body composition you achieve during marathon or half-marathon training. This requires a little work because most of the grain foods sold in supermarkets and restaurants are made with refined grains, some of which are disguised as whole grains. Most so-called wheat breads, for example, are not whole-grain foods. A typical case is the "9-grain wheat bread" available at Subway restaurants. It may sound wholesome but it contains no whole grain whatsoever. None of the breads at this particular restaurant do. So if you want a sandwich with 100 percent whole wheat bread, you'll have to go elsewhere.

As public demand for whole-grain options increases, however, such options are becoming more widely available. The Rubio's Mexican restaurant chain now offers whole-grain tortillas, for example. With a little awareness and a bit of research you can minimize your consumption of refined grains without going too far out of your way.

8. FATTY MEATS

Meats produced through modern industrial methods (factory farmed and/or highly processed and packaged meats) tend to be fattier and less nutritious than more natural meats that come from animals that are fed a natural diet and allowed to move about while living. These meats also tend to promote weight gain. I recommend that you avoid eating "industrial" meats as much as possible, instead limiting your meat consumption to organic, free-range, and grass-fed products. These products are expensive and not always easy to find. If you can't always afford or find them, then at least try to limit your meat consumption to products that are less than 10 percent fat.

9. SWEETS

Sugar is the number one cause of weight gain. Sugary foods and beverages including candy, desserts, and soft drinks promote weight gain because they are extremely calorie dense and have very low satiety indices. Most of us require the occasional sweet treat to remain happy eaters, but if you're serious about attaining your optimal racing weight you must limit your intake of sugary foods and beverages to no more than the occasional sweet treat.

One particular type of sugar, high-fructose corn syrup, has received a lot of attention lately—none of it positive. While HFCS is processed by the body somewhat differently than other sugars, the real reason it may be contributing more to the obesity epidemic than are other sugars is simply that it is used far more (because it's cheaper). If you make an effort to minimize the amount of HFCS you consume but make no effort to limit your intake of other added sugars (such as dextrose, or table sugar), you won't make much progress toward your ideal racing weight. All added sugars are fattening; high-fructose corn syrup may just be marginally more so.

10. FRIED FOODS

Frying any type of food in oil adds a lot of calories to the food and thus increases its calorie density. For example, a grilled chicken drumstick contains 90 calories. A fried chicken drumstick contains 150 calories. Fried foods promote weight gain more than any other type of food except sweets, and their effects on heart disease risk are even greater. A Spanish study conducted in 2011 found that, in a sample of nearly ten thousand men and women who were tracked for more than six years, those who ate fried food more than four times a week were significantly more likely to become overweight than were those who ate fried food no more than twice a week.

Fried food is very tasty and hard to resist. I can't help but indulge in it every now and then. But you must avoid it as much as willpower enables you to during marathon or half-marathon training, lest you arrive at the starting line with the consequences clinging to your belly and hips. Note that I'm talking specifically about deep frying. "Light" frying such as sautéing and stir-frying are okay.

Frying is almost always done with oils, of course, but oils are not always used for frying. Oil-based salad dressings are not fried, for example. I'll have more to say about oils on page 49.

DIET QUALITY BALANCE

To raise your diet to a sufficient quality level to attain your ideal racing weight without depriving your body of the energy it needs for optimal training or going hungry, all you have to do is follow one rule: eat vegetables more often than fruits, fruits more often than nuts and seeds, fish and lean meats more often than whole grains, whole grains more often than dairy products, dairy products more often than refined grains, refined grains more often than sweets, and sweets more often than fried foods. That's it. Simply biasing your diet toward the higher-quality food categories in this manner will do the job. You can—and indeed should—eat as much as your appetite dictates. As long as you obey this one rule, it won't be too much.

It is not necessary that you eat more veggies than fruits, more fruits than nuts and seeds, and so forth in every single meal and snack. Instead use a weekly timescale. If, at the end of each week, you have eaten vegetables more often than fruit, fruit more often than nuts and seeds, and so on, then you have attained diet quality balance, even if several meals and snacks included no veggies and even if one of your snacks was a serving of french fries.

Strictly speaking, diet quality balance means this: You must eat at least ten servings of vegetables, nine servings of fruit, eight servings of nuts and seeds, seven servings of lean meats and fish, six servings of whole grains, and five servings of dairy for every one serving of fried food, two servings of sweets, three servings of fatty meats, or four serving of refined grains you eat. This *minimum* requirement to achieve diet quality balance is summarized in Table 2.1.

There is some fine print, however. First, there are only two categories of food that you *must* eat: vegetables (including legumes) and fruits. You may choose to eat these two categories alone if you so desire. But unless you have specific preferences or restrictions that stand in the way, I recommend that you also include nuts and seeds, fish and meat, and whole grains in your diet, for the sake of balance. The less you eat of the remaining categories, the better, but nothing is forbidden.

If you choose to follow a vegetarian diet or any other diet that eliminates one or more of the categories of food that I rate as high quality (such as the Paleo diet, which forbids all grains and dairy products), you'll need to make an adjustment to my one rule to ensure that the overall balance of high-quality and low-quality foods in your diet

TABLE 2.1 *MINIMUM REQUIREMENT FOR DIET QUALITY BALANCE*

FOOD CATEGORY	NUMBER OF SERVINGS EATEN IN A GIVEN SPAN OF TIME
Vegetables	10
Fruits	9
Nuts and seeds	8
Fish and lean meats	7
Whole grains	6
Dairy products	5
Refined grains	4
Fatty meats	3
Sweets	2
Fried foods	1

doesn't shift toward the latter. In such cases just be sure that at least forty-five of every fifty-five foods you eat are high-quality foods, as would be the case if you included all ten foods categories in your diet in the balance required by the one rule.

Among the four low-quality food categories, you don't really *have to* eat the higher-ranked ones more often than the lower-ranked ones. In other words, if you eat a fried food in a given span of time, you shouldn't feel compelled to eat sweets at least twice, fatty meats at least three times, and refined grains at least four times within that same span of time. Instead, simply make sure you eat each of the four low-quality food categories less often than any of the six high-quality food categories and try to eat the lowest-ranked low-quality foods least often.

You might be wondering why I don't just forbid consumption of the low-quality food categories altogether, or at least toss them together under the common (and familiar) heading, "Eat sparingly." The reason is that this is completely unnecessary and, in my view, somewhat misleading. Refined grains (regular old spaghetti being an example), fatty meats (hard salami), sweets (blueberry pie), and fried foods (bacon) are not poisonous. They are foods that just happen to be less wholesome than some other foods. There is no reason to believe that including the low-quality foods in your diet in the amounts permitted by my guidelines for diet quality balance will impede your progress toward your ideal racing weight.

If you do the bare minimum required to heed these guidelines, your diet will consist of 82 percent high-quality foods and 18 percent low-quality foods (and only 3.5 percent sweets and less than 2 percent fried foods). Such a diet (which is also more than one-third vegetables and fruits) is drastically healthier than the average person's diet—and even the average runner's diet—and it's just plain good enough. It's also more sustainable and enjoyable than any diet that classifies blueberry pie and bacon as "cheating" could ever be.

The principle of diet quality balance works very well in real-world practice. Thousands of runners have implemented it (primarily in an earlier version called the Diet Quality Score) with great results. Mark Sands, a policeman in Rochester, New York, who started running in

2002, weighed 178 pounds when he began to practice my diet quality guidelines. He lost 24 pounds and set huge PRs for 5 miles, the half marathon, and the marathon (breaking four hours in the latter after years of falling short despite serious training).

It's okay to give yourself a little flexibility in the high-quality food types as well. I mentioned above that veggies and fruits must be consumed more often than any other food types. Among the other four categories of high-quality foods (nuts and seeds, fish and lean meats, whole grains, and dairy products), you don't need to feel wholly obligated to eat more of the higher-ranked ones just because you've eaten a piece of cheese (for example). It is enough to always eat each of these food categories more often than you eat any of the four low-quality food categories. As a general trend, though, you should eat nuts and seeds more often than fish and lean meats, fish and lean meats more often than whole grains, and whole grains more often than dairy products.

If the second rule of the Two-Rule Diet is beginning to sound a bit more complex than its name suggests, fear not. My diet quality guidelines—fine print and all—are concisely summarized in Table 2.2.

When I say that you should eat the higher-quality categories more often, I mean precisely that, and I don't mean that you must eat greater *amounts* of these foods. There are typical portion sizes of each type of food that we normally consume. A handful of nuts is typical, and so, too, are a whole apple and a palm-size piece of fish. In following the one-rule diet, count each normal portion of each food type as one "occasion" of eating it and make sure that at the end of the week you've eaten more apples than handfuls of nuts and more handfuls of nuts than palm-size pieces of fish (for example). You don't need to get caught up in official or recommended serving sizes. Whatever you normally eat counts as a portion or occasion of eating that particular category of food.

In short, use common sense. If you have a single piece of lettuce and a single slice of tomato on a sandwich, I would count that as half a vegetable portion, not a full one. If you freak out one evening and eat four chocolate chip cookies, I would count that as two portions of sweets.

TABLE 2.2 *SUMMARY OF DIET QUALITY GUIDELINES*

FOOD CATEGORY	QUALITY RANKING	QUALITY ZONE	EATING GUIDELINES
Vegetables	1	High	Eating vegetables is mandatory. On a weekly basis, eat them more frequently than any other food category.
Fruits	2	High	Eating fruits is mandatory. On a weekly basis, eat them more frequently than any other food category except vegetables.
Nuts and seeds	3	High	Eating nuts and seeds is recommended but optional. If you do eat them, eat them at least more often (on a weekly basis) than any category of low-quality food and ideally more often than fish and lean meats, whole grains, and dairy products as well.
Fish and lean meats	4	High	Eating fish and lean meats is recommended but optional. If you do eat them, eat them at least more often (on a weekly basis) than any category of low-quality food and ideally more often than whole grains and dairy products as well.
Whole grains	5	High	Eating whole grains is recommended but optional. If you do eat them, eat them at least more often (on a weekly basis) than any category of low-quality food and ideally more often than dairy products as well. If you're a high-mileage runner you may eat grains more often than nuts and seeds and fish and lean meats.
Dairy products	6	High	Eating dairy products is recommended but optional. If you do eat them, eat them more often (on a weekly basis) than any category of low-quality food.
Refined grains	7	Low	Refined grains are not prohibited but should be generally avoided. If you do eat them, make sure you eat them less often than any category of high-quality food.
Fatty meats	8	Low	Fatty meats are not prohibited but should be generally avoided. If you do eat them, make sure you eat them less often than any category of high-quality food and ideally less often than refined grains as well.
Sweets	9	Low	Sweets are not prohibited but should be generally avoided. If you do eat them, make sure you eat them less often than any category of high-quality food and ideally less often than refined grains and fatty meats as well.
Fried foods	10	Low	Fried foods are not prohibited but should be generally avoided. If you do eat them, make sure you eat them less often than any category of high-quality food and ideally less often than refined grains, fatty meats, and sweets as well.

MORE ON WHOLE GRAINS

The food category whose position on my quality continuum may be most alarming to you is that of whole grains. Am I really suggesting that you have to eat nuts and seeds more often than whole grains? The reason whole grains are ranked lower than nuts and seeds and fish and lean meats on the diet quality continuum is that, while whole grains are healthy, individuals who exclude whole grains from their diet are likely to be a little leaner than those who exclude either of the other two. Lots of athletes get good results from the currently popular Paleo diet, which excludes whole grains.

If you train heavily, it's okay to move whole grains up the continuum. Runners who train five hours a week or less should generally try to eat nuts and seeds and fish and lean meat (unless they're vegetarian) more often than they eat whole grains. Runners whose average training load is ten hours a week or greater may eat whole grains more often than they do nuts and seeds and fish and lean meat. If you routinely train more than five hours a week but less than ten, your frequency of whole-grain consumption can be about equal to that of your intake of nuts and seeds and fish and lean meat.

The most familiar whole grains are whole wheat, whole oats, brown rice, and corn flour. You can't go wrong with any of these, but there are lots of other options with different tastes and nutrient profiles to give your palate and your body some welcome variety. Following are five alternative whole grains to try. Most can be found at your local natural foods market.

Amaranth: Amaranth seeds have a creamy consistency when cooked, and an earthy taste. Amaranth is among the most fiber-rich and protein-rich grains.

Buckwheat: Also called kasha, buckwheat has a strong, distinctive taste and is rich in the phytonutrient rutin.

Quinoa: Quinoa provides one of the broadest amino acid spectrums in the plant kingdom and is appreciated for its nutty taste.

Spelt: Similar to wheat, spelt contains more protein, fiber, magnesium, selenium, and niacin than its close grain cousin. It has a chewy consistency when cooked, and a light sweetness on the tongue.

Teff: Teff cooks into a porridgelike consistency and has a slightly malty taste. It's a great source of iron, calcium, fiber, and B vitamins, among other nutrients.

COMBINATION FOODS

There are lots of foods that belong in more than one category. Use common sense as well in assigning categories to these foods. For example, count ice cream as both a sweet and a dairy product. If you eat a stromboli for lunch, count the crust as a refined grain, the meatballs as a fatty meat, the cheese as a dairy product, and the tomato sauce as half a vegetable portion.

BEVERAGES

Plain or lightly sweetened coffee and tea can be excluded from the diet quality equation. Coffee and tea drinks containing more than 50 calories should be counted as sweets.

Diet soft drinks should be counted as sweets as well. Even though they contain few or no calories, research has shown they fatten us just as much as sugar-filled soft drinks. Each portion of 100 percent vegetable or fruit juice should be counted as half a vegetable or fruit portion. There are those who say these juices are equivalent to whole vegetables and fruits, but they're not. Any type of juice that contains added sugar should be counted as a sweet.

Alcoholic beverages do not need to be classified in any food category or even included in your diet quality balance tallies unless you have more than two in a day. Research has shown that people who consume one or two drinks a day are slightly healthier than those who consume less, while those who consume more than two drinks a day are significantly less healthy than those who consume less. If you have more than two drinks in a day, count them as sweets. All mixed drinks containing sugar (e.g., margaritas) should be counted as sweets.

OILS

Some nutritionists treat oils as a separate category of food. I don't because oils are almost always used in other foods and are seldom consumed plain, so it's more practical to focus on the foods they're used in.

One reason some nutritionists treat oils as a distinct food category is that it helps them to construct a diet with healthy fat guidelines—that is, a diet that includes enough essential fats and not too much saturated fat or total fat. In my view this bottom-up approach (focusing on nutrients instead of foods) is needlessly complicated. You can easily avoid eating too much saturated and total fat without ever thinking about oils per se and instead following my diet quality guidelines. To ensure that you get enough essential fats, take a daily omega-3 fat supplement as described in the preceding chapter.

SAUCES, CONDIMENTS, ENERGY BARS, AND DAIRY ALTERNATIVES

Sauces and condiments can be excluded from your tally, unless they contribute nontrivial amounts of calories to meals or snacks. Examples of this are the mayonnaise in tuna salad and the barbecue sauce on barbecued chicken. In such cases you should add them to any of the low-quality food categories.

Energy bars should be counted as sweets unless they are made primarily with whole grains, nuts, seeds, and/or real fruit, in which case you may count them as half-servings of whole grains, nuts, etc.

If you are lactose intolerant or do not eat dairy foods for any other reason you may count any dairy alternatives in your diet as dairy foods. Examples are hemp milk, tofu cheese, and coconut yogurt.

KEEPING COUNT

Remember, maintaining diet quality balance does not require that you eat more vegetables than fruits, more fruits than nuts and seeds, and so forth every single day. As I suggested earlier, given the diversity of food categories this would not be a reasonable expectation. Instead I recommend that you take it week by week; keep a running total of the number of foods of each type you've eaten and make sure that by the end of each week you've eaten more vegetables than fruits and so forth.

At the back of this book you will find a training and nutrition journal that is formatted to allow for easy week-by-week tracking of your frequency of consumption of each food category. You're probably accustomed to logging your workouts. I urge you to use this journal or something like it to log your nutrition as well. It is no less important to your success in marathons and half-marathons.

In the next chapter I will provide more specific examples of how to eat for diet quality balance and meet your individual carbohydrate needs simultaneously.

PRACTICING THE TWO-RULE DIET

When Deena Kastor (then Deena Drossin) was eleven years old she fell in love twice: first with running and then with cooking. At first she thought of her athletic and culinary passions as completely separate, but as she grew older they converged. At the University of Arkansas, Kastor spent what little free time she had outside of classes and track practice reading cooking magazines, wandering the aisles of grocery stores, and sweating over a hot oven. One benefit of these extracurricular activities was that Kastor ate much better than the average college student did. This may be one reason she was an eight-time NCAA All-American at Arkansas.

Kastor went on to achieve even greater success as a professional runner. She set American records in the marathon and half marathon that still stand, won the Chicago and London Marathons, earned a pair of World Cross Country Championships bronze medals, won numerous national championship titles, and, most memorably, took home a bronze medal from the 2004 Olympic Marathon. Throughout her stellar career Kastor was fueled largely by her own cooking and she always believed that her love of food preparation was a major contributor to her success.

I think she's right. There's a difference between nutrition knowledge and food knowledge. Having nutrition knowledge is great, but we don't eat nutrition—we eat food. To eat well it is necessary to translate nutrition knowledge into food knowledge. This is where people who like to cook have an advantage. Women and men who are comfortable in the kitchen tend to stock their refrigerator and cupboards with better foods, include greater variety in their diet, rely less on fast and processed foods, and therefore eat healthier than do people who don't cook, regardless of their level of nutrition knowledge.

I'm not saying you have to be a world-class chef (I'm not) or prepare a complicated dinner every night (I don't) to eat healthily. I'm just trying to make the point that eating well comes down to eating good food. And the purpose of this chapter is to help you do just that.

As you've seen, there are just two basic rules you need to follow in your everyday diet as a runner. First, you need to consume enough carbohydrate to get the most out of your training. In addition to this, you need to maintain diet quality balance to shed excess body fat and get down to your optimal racing weight. Naturally, you must heed these two rules simultaneously in your diet. To do this successfully you will need to base your diet on meals and snacks that include lots of high-carbohydrate, high-quality foods but not so exclusively that variety—or enjoyment—is sacrificed.

"I believe you can eat anything you want," Deena Kastor told me back in 2003. "It's okay to satisfy your junk food desires, as long as you fill up mainly on healthy foods."

The process of bringing your eating habits in line with the Two-Rule Diet will not take place in a vacuum. You already have a particular way of eating that you must now modify to some extent for the sake of your running. There are well-defined eating customs in our society. By tradition we eat three meals a day and perhaps one or more between-meal snacks as well. These meals have traditional compositions; most people don't want sushi for breakfast or oatmeal for dinner even if they can be convinced that these choices make nutritional sense. Fortunately, you can elevate your diet quality and get enough carbohydrate to support optimal training without flouting such cultural conventions. In this chapter I will present a selection of normal, recognizable foods to eat for breakfast, lunch, dinner, and snacks that will enable you to consistently meet your diet quality requirement and your carbohydrate needs. These meals and snacks are offered merely as suggestions and guidelines and should not be considered mandatory. There are plenty of other foods you can use to attain diet quality balance and meet your carbohydrate needs. Feel free to go with your personal preferences.

BREAKFAST

What you eat for breakfast and even when you eat it should be dependent upon when you normally run. If you run soon after waking up in the morning you cannot eat a full breakfast before heading out the door. Doing so would result in stomach discomfort as the bolus of food in your gut was jostled around, and it would also rob your working muscles of blood flow as blood was shunted to your gastrointestinal tract to support digestion.

On the other hand, running on a completely empty stomach after an overnight fast would compromise your run in a different way. When you start any run your muscles initially rely predominantly on blood glucose for fuel. The blood glucose level is kept from falling by the breakdown of liver glycogen. During sleep the central nervous system is kept functioning by blood glucose, which, as during exercise, is maintained from liver glycogen stores. These stores are 50 percent depleted when you get out of bed in the morning. If you wake up and run without eating first you are likely to feel sluggish and perform suboptimally since your muscles' go-to energy source is severely compromised.

So it's important that you eat or drink *something* before you run, even if you start running within ten or fifteen minutes of waking up. That something should be mostly carbohydrate, to provide a second reservoir from which your blood glucose concentration can be maintained. This high-carb snack should come in a form that is easily digested and it should be large enough to make a difference in how you feel and perform yet small enough not to cause stomach discomfort.

A banana, a packet of energy gel, or a small bowl of nonfat yogurt will do the job. Your first full meal of the day can wait until you return from your workout.

If you run at any other time of day besides first thing in the morning it's fine to eat a full breakfast soon after waking. Regardless of whether you eat this meal before or after your run, it should be high in carbohydrate, as runners need their breakfast to make a significant contribution toward meeting their daily carbohydrate needs. Many commonly eaten breakfast foods, such as cold cereal and bagels, contain large amounts of carbohydrate. Just be sure to choose those that are made with 100 percent whole grains.

Because a runner's approach to breakfast is dependent on his or her running schedule, it's worthwhile to consider the best time of day to run. Should you run early in the morning? In the afternoon? Both?

Studies have shown that most people perform better and also feel more comfortable when they exercise in the afternoon. Other research, however, has shown that exercise performance improves most at the specific time of day when workouts are habitually performed. If you always work out in the afternoon your afternoon exercise performance will increase more than your morning workout performance. And if you always work out in the morning your morning workout performance will improve more than your afternoon workout performance.

Most marathons and half marathons take place early in the morning. Therefore you'll want to do at least some of your workouts in the early morning so that your race performances aren't compromised by a lack of specific physiological adaptation to exercising at that time of day. If you're normally an afternoon exerciser, breaking from that habit once or twice a week should suffice to ensure that you don't put yourself at a disadvantage in morning races. Go ahead and do all of your runs in the morning if that's what works best for your schedule. Of course, many elite runners train twice a day, which gives them the best of both worlds: specific adaptation to running in the morning, plus the benefits of feeling and performing better in afternoon workouts.

Some runners have little appetite early in the morning and prefer to wait at least a couple of hours after waking before they eat anything. If you currently wait until midmorning or later to eat your first meal of the day you might want to consider experimenting with eating earlier to see if you can get comfortable with it. Not only will this make it easier for you to meet your daily carbohydrate needs but it might also help you reach your optimal racing weight. Several large-scale studies have associated regular breakfast skipping with higher levels of body fat. One theory is that eating early in the day reduces appetite through the remainder of the day. But people who eat breakfast typically eat more total calories in a day than do people who skip breakfast. Because these extra calories aren't making breakfast eaters fatter, another theory holds that eating breakfast tends to increase activity levels the rest of the day.

If you choose to persist in the habit of delaying your first meal of the day, then you probably should also be an afternoon runner, or at least reserve your harder runs for the afternoons, as you're unlikely to have enough energy to perform optimally in the morning.

TOP 5 BREAKFASTS FOR RUNNERS

Your breakfast should not only help you meet your daily carbohydrate needs but give you a good start toward meeting your diet quality goals as well. Fruits and vegetables are less often included in breakfast menus than grains. I urge you to eat at least one portion of fruit or veggies in every breakfast because doing so will make it easier for you to attain diet quality balance by the end of each week.

Each of my "Top 5 Breakfasts for Runners" contains at least one portion of fruit or veggies. You can get another half portion by drinking a glass of fruit or vegetable juice (unless your breakfast is a fruit smoothie or a smoothie with leafy greens, which already contains fruit juice or veggies).

BREAKFAST WRAP

Here's an easy breakfast wrap that provides one portion each of whole grains, vegetables, and lean meat (the egg). The carbohydrate content depends on its size and the exact ingredients. A wrap that's made with a 10-inch whole wheat tortilla, one egg, ½ cup of pinto beans, 1 cup of veggies, and 1 tablespoon of avocado supplies a total of 64 g of carbs.

continues ...

BREAKFAST WRAP [CONTINUED]

INGREDIENTS (note that veggie amounts
   are approximate—feel free to experiment)
½ onion, diced
½ red bell pepper, seeded and diced
½ cup spinach (or other veggies to your liking), diced
½ cup precooked or canned black beans or
   pinto beans (drain and rinse if canned)
1 large egg
1 whole wheat soft tortilla
Optional: avocado (diced), cheese, and hot sauce, to taste

In a skillet over medium heat, sauté the onion, pepper, and spinach. Stir in the beans to heat them. Crack the egg into a bowl, whip it briefly, and add it to the veggies and beans. Heat a dry skillet; place the tortilla on the skillet for 5 seconds, flip it, and toss it onto a plate. Scoop the mixture of veggies, beans, and egg onto the tortilla and wrap it up to eat. Add avocado, cheese, and hot sauce, if desired.

CEREAL WITH MILK AND FRUIT

Cold breakfast cereals vary widely in quality. The highest-quality cereals are made with whole grains and contain little added sugar. Some also contain extra goodies, such as seeds, nuts, and dried fruit. The lowest-quality cereals are made with refined grains and contain lots of added sugar. I suggest that you buy only cereals whose first ingredient is some type of whole grain and buy no cereal that lists any form of sugar among its first two ingredients. Among the products that meet these criteria are Bob's Red Mill Granola, Cheerios, Cinnamon Puffins, Ezekiel 4:9 Organic Golden Flax, Fiber One Honey Clusters, Kashi GoLean, Nature's Path Flax Plus Flakes, Post Grape-Nuts Flakes, Post Raisin Bran, and Quaker Oatmeal Squares.

You can increase the quality of any cereal and improve the quality of your breakfast by adding fresh fruit to the bowl. Blueberries, strawberries, and sliced bananas taste good in most cereals. Add a generous amount of fruit to make it count as one whole fruit portion.

Use whole milk if you prefer the taste or prefer dairy products that are minimally processed. Use skim milk if you're more concerned about fat. Yogurt is also a great option. And if you don't drink cow's milk at all, use a nondairy option such as soy, almond, or hemp milk.

A bowl of healthy cereal with milk and fresh fruit counts as one portion of whole grain, one portion of dairy, and one portion of fruit, for diet quality monitoring purposes. The total contribution toward your daily carbohydrate needs depends on the specific cereal you choose, the kind of milk, and the portions. Two cups of Cheerios with 1 cup of whole milk and about ½ cup of fresh blueberries provides 58 g of carbs. A 12-ounce glass of orange juice on the side adds 35 g of carbohydrate and another half-portion of fruit.

FRUIT AND/OR VEGGIE SMOOTHIE

By drinking a smoothie for breakfast you can get three or even four servings of fruit or veggies in your body right out of the gate and get a strong start toward diet quality balance. Smoothies aren't just for fruit: You can also add carrot juice, greens, or other veggies to the blender to take a step toward your vegetable quota while still drinking something that tastes sweet and fruity. For an even more balanced meal, toss in a couple of scoops of yogurt or your favorite protein powder.

Fruit smoothies deliver a lot of carbohydrate in a form that is easily digested. You may even be able to use a small smoothie to fuel an early-morning run without risk of stomach upset. The following smoothie contains 70 g of carbs and also counts as four portions of fruit and one of vegetables.

QUICK BREAKFAST SMOOTHIE
1 cup orange juice
1 banana
1 cup raw spinach
½ cup frozen blueberries
½ cup frozen strawberries

Place all the ingredients into the blender, press go, and voilà!—a quick, high-energy breakfast is served. You can play around with this recipe, substituting your favorite fruits or veggies, as well as dairy or nondairy milk or different flavors of juices.

OLD-FASHIONED OATMEAL WITH FRUIT AND NUTS

Old-fashioned oatmeal is a terrific source of carbohydrate and also a welcoming host to the flavors of other high-quality foods: namely, fresh or dried fruit and nuts. Fresh apple slices, raisins, almond slivers, walnuts, and pecans are popular additions. The following mixture provides 72 g of carbohydrate and one portion each of whole grains, fruit, nuts and seeds, and (alas) sweets.

½ cup whole oats
½ cup apple, cored and diced
¼ cup chopped pecans
2 tablespoons pure maple syrup

Combine 1 cup of water and the oats in a pot and bring to a boil. Reduce the heat and let the oats simmer until most of the water has been absorbed. Remove from the heat and pour into a bowl. Add the apple, pecans, and maple syrup and stir.

WHOLE WHEAT BAGEL SANDWICH

You can have a breakfast sandwich without having an Egg McMuffin. Toast a whole wheat bagel; stack one cooked egg, one slice of Cheddar cheese, one fat tomato slice, and a few slices of avocado between the bagel halves; and you have a healthy breakfast that delivers 62.5 g of carbs and one portion each of whole grains, lean meat, dairy, and vegetables.

SNACKS

To snack or not to snack: that is the question. Some nutrition experts discourage snacking on the grounds that most of us eat too many calories even without munching between meals. Other nutrition experts encourage healthy snacking as part of a "grazing" approach to diet that is based on the belief that eating small amounts of food frequently throughout the days boosts metabolism, prevents weight gain, maintains more consistent energy levels, and prevents blood-sugar "crashes."

My view is that snacking is good for some people and bad for others. Most nonrunners are probably better off not snacking. They don't burn enough calories to justify eating outside of regular meals and the supposed benefits of increased metabolism, improved blood sugar regulation, and so forth are not supported by science. Runners are more likely to need snacks to meet their elevated energy and carbohydrate needs. Hunger between meals, sluggishness in workouts, and a daily carbohydrate intake that falls short of your calculated needs are indications that you may need to snack.

No matter how often you eat, you don't eat often enough that you can waste one of your day's eating occasions on unhealthy foods, which will only force you to eat extra "cleanly" over the next few days to ensure that your diet quality balance is right before the end of the week. I encourage you to approach snacks as chances to eat more of the food categories you aren't getting enough of in your meals.

TOP 5 SNACKS FOR RUNNERS

These five snacks are not the only acceptable between-meal hunger-killers for runners. Whole wheat pretzels, for example, are a good source of carbs, while high-quality jerky is a good source of lean protein. But the snacks on my list provide the best mix of carbohydrate and diet quality.

VEGGIES AND DIP

Diet quality balance requires that you eat vegetables more frequently than you eat anything else. Adhering to this rule necessitates that you continuously look for chances to eat veggies. Snacking on veggies is one good option. A handful of broccoli crowns dipped in ranch salad dressing provides 6 g of carbs and, of course, counts as one vegetable portion. A handful of baby carrots dipped in old-fashioned (just peanuts and salt) peanut butter provides 9 g of carbs and counts as one vegetable portion and one portion of nuts and seeds.

Be sure to choose (or prepare) high-quality dips, such as dressings without sugar and preservatives, and use them lightly. The vegetables should predominate in these snacks.

WHOLE FRUIT

Why make snacking complicated? A nice, ripe, in-season pear or peach gives you one portion of the second-ranked category of food in the diet quality continuum and delivers a large dose of carbohydrate. The precise amount of carbohydrate varies greatly by fruit type and size. One medium-size pear contains 26 g of carbs, while a large peach contains 15 g.

YOGURT WITH FRUIT

As I mentioned earlier, yogurt has some great health benefits. Some yogurts are healthier than others, however. Most yogurts contain added sugar, which I find unnecessary because yogurt contains lactose sugar naturally. If you choose to snack on yogurt, I encourage you to purchase unflavored yogurt without added sugar and sweeten it—while also raising the snack's diet quality—by adding your own fresh fruit to it. Check the label on yogurt you purchase. You can also purchase a larger tub and customize your yogurt with each serving.

As with other dairy products, choose a low-fat or nonfat yogurt if you're concerned about fat intake; choose a whole-milk yogurt if you prefer foods in more natural forms. You're also free to choose between American-style yogurt and Greek yogurt, which has more protein and less carbohydrate.

An 8-ounce serving of whole Greek yogurt with a handful of fresh raspberries mixed in provides 12 g of carbohydrate and counts as one dairy portion and one fruit portion.

NUTS, SEEDS, AND/OR DRIED FRUIT

Nuts, seeds, and dried fruit are nature's snack foods. Many different kinds of nuts, seeds, and dried fruits are good for snacking and the options are even greater when you combine them. Be sure to read product labels carefully, however, and avoid those with added sugar, preservatives, and other ingredients besides nuts, fruit, seeds, and natural flavorings. One of my favorite combinations is Eden Foods' All Mixed Up, which contains roasted almonds, pumpkin seeds, dried cherries, and raisins. One official serving provides 7 g of carbs, but I usually eat about a serving and a half and count it as one portion of nuts and seeds and a half-portion of fruit.

SNACK BAR

Energy bars and snack bars are an unfortunate crutch for many runners. Almost all of these foods are calorie dense without being particularly nutrient dense and contain a lot of added sugar. But I recognize that bars are convenient and tasty, they squelch hunger very effectively, and many runners will eat them no matter what I say. If you depend on bars, at least purchase one of the few that are relatively high-quality foods made primarily with seeds, nuts, whole grains, and real fruit. Don't fall for those whose labels throw lots of healthy-sounding words at you ("organic," "raw food") while listing disguised sugars ("brown rice syrup") as their first ingredient. Avoid bars with a lot of ingredients—the best ones are simple, with a handful of quality components.

The ingredients list of my favorite snack bar reads as follows: "Sprouted organic flaxseeds, organic apricot, organic raisins, organic date, organic lime juice." That's the kind of snack bar you should eat. This particular product delivers 7 g of carbohydrate per serving and I count it as one portion of nuts and seeds and a half-portion of fruit.

LUNCH

The traditional American lunch is a sandwich, a bag of potato chips, and a can of soda or some other sweetened drink. There's a fair amount of carbohydrate in such a meal but not much quality. The major challenge that runners accustomed to American-style lunches face in the midday meal is to consume a meaningful amount of fruits and/or vegetables to contribute toward their diet quality balance.

There's nothing inherently wrong with sandwiches. I myself eat them fairly regularly. When I do eat a sandwich for lunch I usually maximize the quality by using whole-grain bread; including veggies in the sandwich; eating a small salad, some vegetable soup, or baby carrots with ranch dressing as a side item; and washing it all down with a glass of Spicy Hot V8 juice. There's a lot of repetition in these meals, but I don't sweat it. Variety in the diet is somewhat overrated. It's a heck of a lot better to eat the same healthy lunch day after day than to have a different unhealthy lunch each day. And it isn't that hard to mix it up. You can choose different veggies for the sandwich, add healthy flavor to them with a variety of spreads (mustard, hummus, tapenade, nut butters, and all-fruit spreads), try new soups, and eat in-season fruits (e.g., oranges in winter, watermelon in summer) for dessert. Otherwise, rely more on your dinners for variety.

One easy way to increase both the variety and quality of your lunches is to have dinner—that is, leftovers, for lunch. I do this often. High-carbohydrate, high-quality dinner options are almost unlimited. Microwaving the latest kitchen creation of my wife, Nataki, at noon the next day is a convenient (perhaps even lazy) way to ensure that my midday meals are as helpful to my running as my evening meals.

TOP 5 LUNCHES FOR RUNNERS

Sandwiches and soups are traditional lunch foods that can easily contribute both the carbs and the quality you need as a runner training for a marathon or half marathon. If you have a smaller appetite, choose one or the other each day. If you have an appetite like mine, have both. Or a burrito!

CHICKEN CAESAR SALAD WRAPS

As I said, there's nothing wrong with a good sandwich, but wraps have one advantage, which is that you can fit a whole salad's worth of vegetables inside them. Here's one example.

    2 cups romaine lettuce, which has been
        washed and broken into bite-size pieces
    2 tablespoons Caesar salad dressing
    1 chicken breast, cut into strips
    2 (8-inch) whole wheat soft tortillas

Place the lettuce in a bowl and mix in the salad dressing. Place a skillet over medium-high heat and lightly coat it with olive oil. Add the chicken strips and stir occasionally until they are fully cooked (about 4 minutes). Remove the chicken from the skillet and add to the salad mixture. Heat the tortillas on the skillet for

continues ...

CHICKEN CAESAR SALAD WRAP [CONTINUED]

10 seconds per side. Spoon half of the chicken salad mixture onto the center of each wrap and fold.

Two wraps provide 45 g of carbs and count as one portion each of whole grains, lean meat, and vegetables.

SPLIT PEA SOUP

There's nothing like a good homemade soup, but certain canned soups are just as nutritious and almost as tasty, while being much easier to prepare. For example, Amy's brand Split Pea Soup contains the same ingredients you would put in your own homemade version: filtered water, organic green split peas, organic onions, organic celery, organic carrots, organic basil, sea salt, organic garlic, "spices," and organic black pepper. One can contains 2 cups of soup and provides 38 g of carbs. Count it as one vegetable portion (even if you eat half a can with a sandwich). Want to get even more veggies in? Add fresh vegetables to your canned soup.

BUTTERNUT SQUASH SOUP

Some soups are best made at home instead of bought ready made. Butternut squash soup is one of them. Most canned and boxed squash soups contain some form of added sugar and a lot more oil than the recipes for homemade soups require. Here's a quick and easy recipe for butternut squash soup. Be sure to use one of the more wholesome brands of vegetable stocks, such as Pacific Natural Organic Vegetable Broth, which are made without sweeteners, preservatives, and other stuff you wouldn't put in a homemade stock.

1 butternut squash, peeled, seeded, and cut into small cubes
1 yellow onion, diced
32 ounces vegetable stock
2 tablespoons olive oil
Salt and freshly ground black pepper

Preheat the oven to 450°F. Place the squash and onion on a baking sheet lined with aluminum foil. Drizzle with the olive oil and sprinkle salt and pepper over the veggies. Bake until a fork passes easily through the squash, about 45 minutes. Pour the stock into a large pot and bring to a simmer. Stir in the veggies. Remove from heat, pour the mixture into a blender, and puree.

A large bowl (2 cups) of this soup provides 38 g of carbs and counts as one vegetables serving.

TURKEY (OR OTHER) SANDWICH

Who doesn't like a nice turkey sandwich for lunch? Vegetarians, for starters. But for the rest of us, this American lunch classic can be the centerpiece of a very runner-friendly lunch. My favorite version of the classic includes whole wheat sourdough bread, mustard, avocado, organic smoked turkey breast sliced fresh at the deli counter, tomato, lettuce, and onion. One sandwich made with Vermont Bread Company brand Whole Wheat Sourdough bread and three slices of turkey provides about 39 g of carbs. If you pile the veggies high enough you can go ahead and count them as one full vegetable portion.

Of course, it doesn't have to be turkey. Chicken breast, lean roast beef, and extra-lean ham are among the alternatives that count as lean meats. And if you are a vegetarian, swap out the meat for a fleshy vegetable such as roasted eggplant or portobello mushroom.

CHICKEN, BEAN, AND VEGGIE BURRITO

This tasty, well-balanced "Mexican sandwich" provides 54 g of carbs and counts as one portion each of whole grains, lean meat, and vegetables.

> 3 ounces chicken breast, cut into strips
> ½ cup precooked or canned black beans
>   (drain and rinse if canned)
> ½ cup (total) seeded and sliced green and red bell peppers
> ¼ cup diced onion
> 3 tablespoons pureed avocado
> ¼ diced tomato
> 2 (8-inch) whole wheat soft tortillas

Place a skillet over medium-high heat and lightly coat with olive oil. Place the chicken in the skillet. Add the beans and veggies. Cook, stirring occasionally, until the chicken is fully cooked (about 5 minutes). Remove the burrito filling from the skillet. Heat the tortillas on the skillet for 10 seconds per side. Place half of the burrito filling on the center of each tortilla and fold.

DINNER

Dinner is an important meal because it represents your last chance (unless you eat an evening snack) to attain your carbohydrate intake and diet quality goals for the day. It's best to know where you stand in relation to these goals as you plan your dinner so you can prepare it accordingly.

Your goal of getting the greatest possible benefit as a runner from your suppers will be greatly assisted if you cook for yourself. When you make your own dinners you have total control over what you put in your body and nothing stands in the way of your getting the carbs and quality you need. It doesn't have to be hard. Very simple recipes can be just as healthy as more complex ones. You can start with just one or two meals that you eat over and over and then gradually expand your repertoire. You can also rely on the increasing number of shortcuts to healthy home cooking that are available, such as preseasoned wild-caught fish fillets from your local fish market and single-serving portions of precooked whole-grain brown rice from your local natural foods grocer. Precut fruits and veggies are also great time and sanity savers.

TOP 5 DINNERS FOR RUNNERS

In addition to being your last chance to meet the day's carbohydrate and diet quality targets, dinner is your best chance to increase the variety of your diet. There are only so many breakfast and lunch menus you can cycle through without making the planning and preparation of these meals burdensome. It's easier to include a much broader spectrum of foods in your evening meals. By no means should the five dinner menus presented here be the only five you eat, despite my use of the "Top 5" label. And again, you may also increase the variety of your lunches by eating dinner leftovers at noontime.

WHOLE WHEAT CAPELLINI WITH SPINACH PESTO SAUCE

There's a reason pasta is traditionally served at marathon "carbo-loading" dinners. Two ounces of whole wheat capellini (a.k.a. angel hair pasta) delivers 42 g of carbohydrate. A realistic 6-ounce portion of capellini stuffs 126 g of carbs into your body! Boil 1 cup of fresh spinach and mix it into some jarred or homemade pesto sauce and you've added 10 g of carbs and a vegetable portion to your meal, which, of course, also counts as a portion of whole grains. Round out the meal with a small salad for an extra veggie portion.

GRILLED TUNA STEAK, AMARANTH, AND KALE

There are lots of simple marinade recipes you can use to add flavor and a little carbohydrate to fresh ahi tuna steaks. Here's one:

MARINADE
¼ cup orange juice
¼ cup soy sauce
2 tablespoons olive oil
1 tablespoon freshly squeezed lemon juice
2 tablespoons chopped fresh parsley

continues ...

1 clove garlic, minced
½ teaspoon chopped fresh oregano
½ teaspoon freshly ground black pepper
4 tuna steaks

Combine all of the marinade ingredients in a casserole dish. Reserve several tablespoons of the marinade separately in a small bowl or cup, for basting (a
basic food safety tip), then place the tuna steaks in the casserole dish and immediately flip them so both sides are coated. Let the steaks sit in the marinade
for 30 minutes while you prepare the grill. Cook the steaks for about 5 minutes
per side, basting them occasionally with the reserved marinade. Serving size
is one steak.

Amaranth makes a great side dish for this meal. A half-cup of amaranth provides
62 g of carbs. It is prepared much like rice: add it to boiling water and allow
it to simmer for about 20 minutes. Seasoning can be as basic as a little sea
salt or you can fancy it up a bit with one of the many recipes available online.

Kale adds a vegetable portion to this meal, which also counts as one portion of fish
and one portion of whole grains. One cup of chopped, boiled kale delivers 7
g of carbs. Add flavor by mixing in a little minced garlic and balsamic vinegar.

SALMON BURGER WITH SWEET POTATO WEDGES AND SPINACH SALAD

1 pound fresh salmon
1 cup chopped red onion
¼ cup sliced fresh basil
¼ teaspoon salt
¼ teaspoon freshly ground black pepper
1 tablespoon hot pepper sauce
1 egg white
4 whole wheat sesame buns, lightly toasted

Chop up the salmon and add it to a bowl containing the chopped red onion, basil,
salt, pepper, and hot pepper sauce. Mix everything together, add the egg
white to the bowl and stir thoroughly. Shape the salmon mixture into four equal-
size patties and cook them in a frying pan with a little oil over medium heat
for 3 minutes per side. Serve each on a lightly toasted bun.

You can't very well serve such a fancy burger with regular french fries. It has to be
sweet potato fries—preferably home cooked. They're easy: Combine a couple
of tablespoons of olive oil and a pinch each of brown sugar, grated nutmeg,
salt, pepper, and fresh thyme in a bowl. Cut one or more sweet potatoes into
small wedges and coat each wedge in the mixture.

Preheat your oven to 400°F and bake the sweet potatoes for 1 hour, turning them
after 30 minutes.

continues ...

SALMON BURGER WITH SWEET POTATO WEDGES [CONTINUED]

Round out the meal with a spinach salad with your choice of veggies and dressing. Assuming you eat about 4 ounces of sweet potato and 1 cup of spinach, this meal provides 58 g of carbs. It also counts as two vegetable portions, one whole-grain portion, and one fish portion.

TOFU AND VEGETABLE STIR FRY

Dining alone? Vegetarian? Here's an easy-to-prepare meatless stir-fry for one.

    ½ cup raw brown rice
    1 tablespoon sunflower or safflower oil
    2 cups bok choy
    ¼ cup baby corn
    ¼ cup seeded and sliced bell pepper
    ¼ cup mushrooms
    4 ounces tofu, cubed
    2 tablespoons soy sauce

Bring 1 cup of water to a boil in a pot and add the brown rice. Cover and reduce the heat, allowing the rice to simmer until water is fully absorbed (40 to 50 minutes). Place a skillet over medium heat and lightly coat it with the oil. Add the bok choy, corn, bell pepper, mushrooms, tofu, and soy sauce and cook until the bok choy is tender. Place the rice on a plate and cover with the stir fry. I count this meal, which contains 35 g of carbs, as two portions of vegetables and one portion of whole grains.

LENTIL STEW

Lentils are a nutritionally balanced food that provide lots of carbs, some protein, fiber, vitamins, and minerals; they also serve as a versatile base for hearty meals for hungry runners. You can make an infinite variety of lentil stews with minimal fuss using a slow cooker. Here's one:

    1 cup lentils, presoaked
    2 cups vegetable or beef stock
    1 cup fresh spinach
    1 chopped tomato
    ½ yellow onion, diced
    1 carrot, sliced
    4 ounces lean kielbasa (optional)

Combine all the ingredients except the spinach in a slow cooker. Turn the setting to MEDIUM and leave for 4½ hours. Add the spinach and cook for 30 minutes more. One large bowl of this lentil stew (with or without meat) will supply about 51 g of carbs. If you want additional carbs (and a portion of whole grains), use a

continues ...

warm slice of fresh whole-grain artisan bread for dipping. The stew itself counts as two vegetable portions and, if you add lean meat, one portion of lean meat.

HITTING YOUR NUMBERS

As a runner in training for a marathon or half marathon you start each day with two basic nutritional goals: to meet your carbohydrate needs as defined in Chapter 1 and to attain diet quality balance as defined in Chapter 2. The only tool you need for the latter is an ongoing record of your food intake by category. Such a tool is built into the integrated training and nutrition journal in the appendix (see page 278). Remember, it's really week by week rather than day by day that diet quality balance must be maintained, so this tool entails weekly tallies of portions eaten by food category.

To ensure that you're meeting your daily carbohydrate needs you also need a tool that tells you how much carbohydrate is contained in the foods you eat. Product labels provide this information, but not everything you eat will be labeled. I use calorieking.com to find the amount of carbohydrate in unlabeled produce, recipes, and restaurant foods.

Following are two examples of one-day meal plans for runners with different carbohydrate needs. The first runner weighs 120 pounds (54.5 kg) and trains for forty minutes per day and therefore (according to Table 1.1, see page 24) needs 3 to 4 g of carbs per kilogram of body weight daily, or 163 to 218 g of carbs in total. The second runner weighs 170 pounds (77.25 kg) and trains for sixty minutes per day and therefore needs 5 to 6 g of carbs per kilogram of body weight daily, or 386 to 463 g of carbs in total.

To demonstrate the versatility of the meals and snacks I've presented, I've given both runners the same base menu. The second runner achieves a much greater total carbohydrate intake with this menu by consuming larger portions and more side items and snacks. You will see in Table 3.1 that both runners adhere to my guidelines for diet quality balance, consuming more vegetables than fruits and so forth, although both consume less than the ideal number of portions of nuts and seeds relative to the other high-quality food categories.

TABLE 3.1 *GUIDELINES FOR DIET QUALITY BALANCE*

RUNNER 1 • WEIGHT: 120 LBS • TRAINING: 40 MIN/DAY
CARBOHYDRATE NEEDS: 163–218 G

MEAL	FOODS	FOOD CATEGORIES	CARBS
BREAKFAST	Breakfast Wrap (page 55) Glass of orange juice	1 whole grain 1 vegetable 1 lean meat 1 fruit	92 g
SNACK	Peach	1 fruit	15 g
LUNCH	Turkey sandwich with cheese	1 whole grain 1 vegetable 1 lean meat 1 dairy	39 g
SNACK	Eden Foods All Mixed Up	1 nuts and seeds ½ fruit	7 g
DINNER	Salmon Burger with Sweet Potato Wedges and Spinach Salad (page 65)	1 whole grain 2 vegetables 1 fish	58 g
TOTAL		4 vegetables 3 fish and lean meats 3 whole grains 2½ fruits 1 dairy 1 nuts and seeds 0 refined grains 0 fatty meats 0 sweets 0 fried foods	196 g

continues ...

By counting carbs, logging the foods you eat by type, and a doing a little planning you can easily end each day having met your carbohydrate needs and each week having met your diet quality requirements. Exactly what you choose to eat for breakfast, lunch, dinner, and any snacks you consume is completely up to you. But if you want the process to be even easier, you can base your marathon or half-marathon training diet on the meals and snacks I've presented in this chapter. I chose them especially to address the diet-quality and carbohydrate needs of runners.

As carbohydrate needs vary widely from one runner to the next, you must put these meals and snacks together in a way that is specific to your own needs. If you train fairly lightly, then your carbohydrate needs will be lower. You may want to include some lower-carb foods

Table 3.1 continued

RUNNER 2 • WEIGHT: 170 LBS • TRAINING: 60 MIN/DAY CARBOHYDRATE NEEDS: 386–463 G			
MEAL	**FOODS**	**FOOD CATEGORIES**	**CARBS**
BREAKFAST	Breakfast Wrap (page 55) Fruit Smoothie (page 57)	4 fruits 2 vegetables 1 whole grain 1 lean meat	134 g
SNACK	Carrot sticks and old-fashioned peanut butter	1 vegetable 1 nuts and seeds	9 g
LUNCH	Turkey sandwich with cheese Split Pea Soup (page 62) 12-ounce glass of V8 Juice	1 whole grain 3 vegetables 1 lean meat 1 dairy	92 g
SNACK	Plain fat-free yogurt with raspberries	1 fruit 1 dairy	24 g
DINNER	Salmon Burger with Sweet Potato Wedges and Spinach Salad (page 65)	1 whole grain 2 vegetables 1 fish	70 g
SNACK	2 bananas	2 fruits	62 g
TOTAL		8 vegetables 7 fruits 3 fish and lean meats 3 whole grains 2 dairy 1 nuts and seeds 0 refined grains 0 fatty meats 0 sweets 0 fried foods	391 g

in your daily meal plans to ensure that you don't eat significantly more carbohydrate than you need. If you train more heavily you can get more carbs by eating larger portions of certain meals or snacks or at least larger portions of the most carb-packed foods within meals.

By practicing the Two-Rule Diet consistently throughout the process of preparing for a marathon or half marathon you will do about 75 percent of what you can do nutritionally to break through the wall on race day. The other 25 percent comes from performance nutrition, which encompasses fueling practice during and immediately after workouts, modifying your diet appropriately during the prerace "taper" period, taking advantage of various nutritional opportunities that are available in the final twenty-four hours before the start horn sounds, and, of course, executing a well-rehearsed nutrition plan during the race.

PART TWO

PERFORMANCE NUTRITION FROM DAY 1 TO RACE DAY

CHAPTER 4

FUELING YOUR WORKOUTS

A good everyday diet is not adequate by itself as nutritional preparation for your best performance in a marathon or half marathon. Meeting your daily carbohydrate needs and maintaining a high-quality diet will push back the wall significantly by making you leaner and lighter and by enabling you to train harder and perform better in workouts. But to get the very most out of your training you must also fuel your body appropriately within workouts.

No workout should be so hard that it puts you at risk of hitting the wall of exhaustion that is so often encountered in longer races. You should, however, regularly experience a moderate to moderately high level of fatigue in workouts. The same fueling practices that you will use in races to maximize your performance (a topic that we will discuss thoroughly in Chapter 7) can also be used in your more challenging workouts to help you run stronger and to thereby enhance the benefit you derive from these training sessions. Fueling your body appropriately in workouts also serves as practice for optimal race nutrition. As we'll see in this chapter, though, there are important differences between workout fueling and race fueling. You'll get the greatest possible benefit from your workout fueling if you approach it somewhat differently than you do race fueling.

WATER AND CARBOHYDRATE

There are two types of nutrition that have the potential to significantly enhance performance when consumed during running: water and carbohydrate. It is no accident that these are the two main ingredients in almost all sports drinks intended for use during exercise. Most sports drinks also contain sodium and other electrolyte minerals to replace some of the same minerals that are lost in sweat, but there is no evidence of any performance-enhancing effect associated with these nutrients. A couple of other nutrients—caffeine and protein—are beneficial in special circumstances. We will look more closely at caffeine and protein in later chapters. But whereas many successful runners never use caffeine or protein for performance enhancement in training, every serious runner takes advantage of water and carbohydrate.

The means by which water and carbohydrate enhance running performance are completely distinct. Water consumption actually does not so much enhance running performance as it prevents the decline in performance that results from dehydration. While sweating has the positive effect of keeping the body cool, it also has the negative effect of reducing blood volume. As blood volume decreases, the heart has to work harder to deliver oxygen to the working muscles and to clear carbon dioxide away from the muscles. This loss of "cardiac efficiency" causes perceived effort to increase, which in turn causes the runner to slow down. Water consumption during running limits the decline in blood volume and maintains cardiac efficiency and performance. A study by English researchers found that men and women were able to run for one hour and forty-three minutes at a moderate intensity when supplied with water compared to only one hour and seventeen minutes when denied water.

Carbohydrate intake enhances running performance in a couple of ways. One of these ways is neurological. When carbohydrate touches the tongue, it activates special receptors that in turn activate a "reward center" in the brain. This triggers a reduction in perceived effort (running starts to feel easier) that allows a runner to run faster without exceeding his or her maximum pain tolerance. Carbohydrate consumption also provides an extra fuel source to the working muscles and thereby increases the maximum speed a runner can sustain over a finite distance without hitting the wall. In one study, runners were able to continue for 20 percent longer in a high-intensity interval workout with carbohydrate supplementation than without.

Because water and carbohydrate enhance running performance through separate mechanisms, their effects are additive. In other words, if you consume both you will perform better than you would if you took in either water or carbohydrate alone. A 1995 study found that runners were able to complete a marathon four minutes faster when they consumed water and carbohydrate together (in a sports drink) than when they drank plain water.

Given the beneficial effects of water intake on running performance, you might think it would be a good idea to drink enough water to completely offset dehydration during every training run you do in preparation for a marathon or half marathon. Not so. Water intake only makes a difference in runs lasting longer than sixty to ninety minutes. Shorter runs don't cause enough dehydration for drinking to matter. What's more, drinking too much may be worse than drinking too little because it causes gastrointestinal discomfort. Also, research has demonstrated that drinking by thirst (which almost never suffices to completely offset dehydration) boosts running performance just as much as drinking to minimize dehydration and with less risk of gastrointestinal distress.

Overdrinking is more common in races than it is during training runs because fluids are abundantly available and many runners believe that drinking as much as possible in races will help them perform better. Indeed, runners have been known to bring the wall on themselves by trying to avoid hitting the wall in this way. Shannon Hays did so in the 2011 Carrollton Festival of Races Marathon. Held in Michigan in late July, the CFR Marathon is always warm and humid. Fearful of becoming dehydrated, Shannon, who worked as a high school Spanish teacher in Suwannee, Georgia, drank much more than normal—too much, it turned out. She developed stomach bloating and nausea and struggled to a 3:56:27 finish—about half an hour off her personal best.

It's the same with carbs. Given the beneficial effects of carbohydrate intake on running performance, you might think it would be a good idea to consume the maximal effective amount of carbohydrate during every training run you do in preparation for a marathon or half marathon. Again, not so. Research has shown that while consuming carbs during exercise does enhance performance in individual workouts, it also interferes with some of the physiological adaptations to training that improve fitness. In other words, carb intake during workouts functions as a kind of metabolic crutch that reduces the benefits of workouts. A runner who relies on carbs too heavily in marathon or half-marathon training therefore risks getting less out of it.

The best approach to fueling your workouts in marathon and half-marathon training is a balanced and measured one. Maximum hydration and heavy reliance on carbohydrate are clearly not the way to go. Yet it is far more common for runners to rely too little than too much on fluid and carb intake during the training process. It is a bit of a hassle, after all, to carry nutrition on a long run. While there is something to be said for unencumbered running, runners pay a price for not lugging the nutrition they need for when they really need it.

There's a "sweet spot" between the all-or-nothing extremes that you'll want to aim for in your workout fueling practices. Locating the sweet spot will not only help you get the most out of your training but will also give you the practice you need to fuel your body optimally in races, where it really counts.

GUIDELINES FOR
FLUID INTAKE DURING TRAINING RUNS

It is difficult for today's runners to imagine running an entire marathon without drinking anything, but it used to be the norm. The first modern marathon was the 1896 Olympic Marathon in Athens, Greece, a race of approximately 25 miles that was won, ironically, by a Greek professional water carrier who drank only a single glass of cognac during the race. While Spyridon Louis's midmarathon brandy sipping did not set a precedent, runners throughout the first half of the twentieth century generally avoided drinking anything during long races because they believed that submitting to their thirst would cause them to become "waterlogged" and slow down. One expert of the time wrote, "Don't get in the habit of drinking and eating in a Marathon race; some prominent runners do, but it is not beneficial."

Drinking was often not even an option in races, where water typically was not provided by race officials and where the provision of water by a runner's supporters was considered unsportsmanlike. Since runners seldom drank in races they tended to eschew drinking in training as well. This was not always easy, especially during long runs undertaken in warm weather. Defying one's thirst in training became a sign of mental toughness. As recently as the 1950s top runners including Jackie Meckler, who set several world records at ultramarathon distances, took pride in their exercise of such self-denial. After his retirement Meckler recalled, "In those days it was quite fashionable not to drink until one absolutely had to."

THE GATORADE EFFECT

How times change. Nowadays the practice of withholding fluid intake for the sake of building mental toughness is rare among runners. Anyone who admitted to doing so would be considered either a self-saboteur or a fool. The great reversal in runners' attitudes toward drinking began in 1965, when the creation of the first sports drink, Gatorade, set off a gold rush of research into the effects of dehydration and fluid intake on endurance performance. Scientists found that dehydration impaired performance, whereas drinking water or Gatorade during prolonged exercise enhanced performance and appeared to aid in thermoregulation (temperature control) as well.

These discoveries brought about a sudden paradigm shift in the hydration practices of distance runners. In 1968 Amby Burfoot won the Boston Marathon without drinking a single drop of water. By 1981 the Boston Athletic Association and other marathon organizers were providing drinks to runners at every other mile, and runners were habitually drinking during their longer training runs without shame.

By the 1990s runners were being encouraged to "drink as much as possible" during longer races and to drink enough to completely offset body fluid losses during workouts. Runners were taught that even a slight degree of dehydration could ruin performance and that anything more than slight dehydration could expose them to a dangerously high risk of heat illness. They were instructed to achieve the desirable goal of zero dehydration by weighing themselves before and after their runs and drinking enough to prevent any weight loss, which typically obligated much more gulping than they thirsted for. In short, the proverbial pendulum had swung completely to the opposite side from where it had started in the late nineteenth century, when runners believed that it was drinking rather than not drinking that ruined performance.

There were two problems with this new, maximalist paradigm of hydration. The first problem was that it was largely a creation of the sports drink industry, which had a vested interest in cajoling runners to guzzle their products. The second problem was that the advice to drink as much as possible was based on flawed science and in practice it often did more harm than good.

Research has consistently shown that runners perform no better when they drink as much as possible than they do when they drink by thirst, even though runners typically replace only 60 to 70 percent of fluid losses when they drink by thirst. Nor does drinking as much as possible keep a runner cooler than drinking by thirst. In fact, the only thing that drinking as much as possible does that drinking by thirst does not is increase the risk of stomach upset.

This was shown in a study conducted by researchers at the University of South Africa. Female runners completed three separate two-hour time trials in a hot environment while drinking a sports drink at three different rates: by thirst; at a moderate rate of 130 ml (about 4 ounces) every fifteen to twenty minutes; and at a high rate of 350 ml (roughly 9 ounces) every fifteen to twenty minutes. The study found no significant differences in finishing times among the three trials. Nor was there any difference in core body temperature. However, during the high-drinking-rate trial, two of the eight subjects suffered severe gastrointestinal distress and had to stop running early.

Scientists are not sure why incomplete rehydration (which is invariably the result of drinking by thirst) works just as well as full rehydration (the result of drinking as much as possible), when unchecked dehydration (the result of not drinking at all) is clearly bad for performance in prolonged runs. One theory is that not all of the weight that a runner loses while running counts toward dehydration. The burning of carbs and fats and the release of water stored with glycogen in the muscles also contribute to weight loss. Hence, when runners replace 60 to 70 percent of the weight they lose in a run with thirst-based drinking, they actually replace all or nearly all of the water lost from body fluid. Another theory is that weight loss during a run decreases the energy cost of running and thus counteracts the negative effect of dehydration on blood volume and cardiac efficiency.

DON'T DISOBEY YOUR THIRST

Whatever the true explanation may be, it is now certain that thirst-based drinking is the best drinking strategy for runners regardless of how much or how little fluid intake results from the use of this strategy and regardless of its effect on dehydration levels. The best proof comes from recent field studies involving elite runners in real races. In a 2012 study, for example, researchers estimated that the male winners of thirteen recent major marathons—all of whom appeared to drink by thirst—consumed only 18.4 ounces of fluid per hour on average and lost 8.8 percent of their body weight, reaching nearly five times the amount of dehydration that is often said to be detrimental to performance. Indeed, the winner of any given race is usually the most dehydrated finisher, because faster runners sweat more and are not able to drink as much. Drinking by thirst, drinking relatively little, and becoming significantly dehydrated clearly do not stop the best runners from winning races.

Whether or not you are in contention to win any races, drinking by thirst is the strategy you should use during races and training runs as well. This approach even works on the hottest days when the sweat rate is highest because runners naturally become thirstier and drink more in warmer environments, so there's no need to consciously adjust your drinking rate based on the weather. Simply listening to your body is always sufficient. Here are the two basic guidelines:

1. There is no need to drink in runs lasting less than one hour. You can if you like as there's no "crutch" effect associated with heavy reliance on fluid intake in the training process as there is with carbohydrate. But because drinking during runs lasting less than an hour does not aid performance and carrying fluid is a slight inconvenience, it is sensible to default to not drinking in these workouts.

2. Always have plenty of fluid available and drink according to your thirst in higher-intensity runs lasting longer than one hour and in all runs lasting longer than two hours. You will perform better and therefore get a greater training effect. In low- and moderate-intensity runs of between one and two hours' duration, drinking probably won't aid your performance but you may be more comfortable if you do drink by thirst in these instances. I typically do not drink in easy runs of less than ninety minutes.

GUIDELINES FOR CARBOHYDRATE INTAKE DURING TRAINING RUNS

Carbohydrate intake is beneficial in runs where your performance might be limited by your body's ability to supply carbs to the working muscles. This limit comes into play in very long runs of moderate intensity, in long runs of moderately high intensity, and in moderately long runs with very high-intensity segments. Examples are an 18-mile endurance run done at a comfortable pace, a 10-mile run that includes 6 miles at half-marathon race pace, and a one-hour run featuring half a dozen two-minute bursts at 5K race pace. In each of these types of runs carbohydrate supplementation is likely to reduce your perceived effort and increase your performance. Shorter and slower runs don't challenge the body enough for carbohydrate consumption to have any meaningful effect. The precise duration and intensity of running that are required to bring carbohydrate supply into play as a performance limiter depend on your individual fitness level. As a general rule, though, if a run is long or fast enough to leave you more than moderately fatigued at the end, then carbohydrate intake would make a difference.

Research indicates that you need 30 g of carbohydrate per hour to attain a measurable performance increase in runs that are hard enough for carbohydrate supply to be a limiting factor. Sixty g per hour is considered to be the minimal rate of carbohydrate intake you need to maximize your performance in the most challenging workouts and in longer races. Further increases in the rate of carbohydrate intake all the way up to 90 g per hour may bring you additional performance benefits in marathons and ultramarathons. Many runners are unable to tolerate such high rates of carbohydrate intake, however.

WHEN CARBS BECOME A CRUTCH

Even when a given run is too short or too low in intensity for its outcome to be influenced by carbohydrate intake, the carbs supplied by a sports drink or energy gel are used preferentially by the muscles. As a result your muscles burn less fat than they would normally. This is not a problem in any single workout. However, runners who rely on supplemental carbohydrate consistently in training expose their muscles to significantly less "fat-burning practice" than their muscles would get if deprived of supplemental carbs. And this *is* a problem, because the degree to which the fat-burning capacity of the muscles improves is a function of the amount of fat-burning practice the muscles get in training. Heavy reliance on supplemental carbohydrate acts as a metabolic crutch that limits fat-burning practice and thus limits improvements in fat-burning capacity. According to research, a previously sedentary person who engages in six weeks of endurance training and fuels every workout with a sports drink is likely to see his or her fat-burning capacity increase by roughly 5 percent. A person who does the same training without carbohydrate is more likely to see his or her fat-burning capacity increase by more than 20 percent. The noted sports nutritionist Bob Seebohar has reported that even in elite runners and triathletes, in whom fat-burning capacity is already highly developed, further increases follow the removal of supplementary carbs from training.

We know that increased fat-burning capacity pushes back the wall and elevates performance in half marathons and marathons. It seems possible, then, that by limiting improvements in fat-burning capacity, reliance on sports drinks and energy gels in training can leave you more likely to hit the wall in races. On the basis of this logic some sports nutritionists advise their clients to leave the drinks and gels at home for all of their workouts and consume carbs only during races, a strategy that is sometimes referred to as train low, race high.

Under the guidance of sports nutritionist Krista Austin, for example, 2004 Olympic Marathon silver medalist and 2009 New York City Marathon winner Meb Keflezighi runs as long as two hours in training without consuming carbohydrate. This habit of deprivation increases his fat-burning capacity to an extremely high level. Then, when he competes in a marathon, he consumes as much carbohydrate as he can tolerate. Research has shown that athletes who train their muscles to rely on fat continue to burn more fat than do other athletes even as their muscles take advantage of the extra carbs supplied to them in a race.

HIGH-LOW TRAINING

Strict carbohydrate deprivation in training has never been shown to enhance racing performance. The few studies that have compared the effects of training with and without supplemental carbohydrate on actual performance have found no advantage. In my view the "train low, race high" method is unnecessarily extreme. I prefer a more moderate approach that I call high-low training. In this approach some workouts are performed with supplemental carbohydrate and some without. Relying on this approach is likely to increase your fat-burning capacity as much as would withholding carbs in every workout. You'll also enjoy the benefits of the performance boost that comes from carbohydrate supplementation in key workouts—benefits that you'll miss out on if you never use sports drinks or energy gels.

The benefits of training with and without carbohydrate are equal even though they are achieved by different means, with carb supplementation enhancing workout performance and carb deprivation enhancing fat-burning capacity. The fact that the benefits of training with and without carbs are achieved by different means indicates that these benefits might be additive, and the two methods complementary. Runners who consume carbs in some workouts and withhold carbs in other workouts may improve more than may runners who do just one or the other because they reap the benefits of enhanced performance in key workouts and increased fat-burning capacity.

Another reason it's best to consume carbs in some workouts is that it serves as practice for carb consumption in races. No one disputes that runners should take in carbs during marathons and, in most cases, half marathons. Practicing with sports drinks and energy gels ahead of races enables you to take in carbs more comfortably in races. Research has shown that while it is not possible to train the gut to absorb more carbs on the run, most runners are able to absorb the same amount of carbs more comfortably after getting some practice. Practicing with sports drinks and gels also gives you the opportunity to develop a personalized fueling plan. Individual runners vary widely in their tolerances and preferences for fluid and carbohydrate intake on the run. The only way you can identify your own tolerances and preferences is through trial and error.

BALANCING "HIGH" AND "LOW" IN TRAINING

If it's better to consume carbs in some workouts and to withhold carbs in other workouts than it is to consume or withhold carbs in every workout, then the obvious next question to ask is what is the ideal balance of "high" and "low" training sessions? This question has not been answered empirically, but my hunch is that it is not important to attain a precise balance. As long as some of your harder workouts are carb-fueled and others are not, your fat-burning capacity will increase more than if you fueled every hard workout with carbs and your fitness will increase more than if you never took advantage of the performance-enhancing power of carbohydrate. An even split down the middle is a good place to start.

You don't need to consume carbohydrate in most runs lasting less than one hour. You may find carb intake beneficial in runs lasting forty-five to sixty minutes that feature significant amounts of running in heart-rate Zone 3 or higher (see Chapter 9 for an explanation of heart-rate training zones). I recommend consuming carbs in roughly half of your runs lasting between one and two hours and consuming carbs in all runs lasting longer than two hours. When you do consume carbs during a run, aim to do so at a rate of at least 30 g per hour (for example, one packet of GU energy gel provides 20 g of carbs). Thirty g per hour will suffice to maximize your performance in most workouts. To maximize your performance in your toughest training sessions you will need to consume at least 60 g of carbs per hour (or at the maximum rate you can comfortably tolerate), as you would do in a race. It is not essential that you actually fuel all such workouts as aggressively as you would a race. But do set aside at least one or two race-simulation workouts in which to practice your race fueling just as you plan to do it in your next event. I'll say more on this topic in the final section of this chapter.

You may have noticed that my guidelines for carbohydrate intake during runs roughly parallel my guidelines for water intake. Conveniently, this means that in most runs in which you consume carbohydrate you will also consume fluid. There are some cases, however, when it will be best to take in one and not the other. Table 4.1 summarizes my guidelines for water and carbohydrate consumption in training runs.

TABLE 4.1 *GUIDELINES FOR WATER AND CARBOHYDRATE INTAKE DURING TRAINING RUNS*

RUN DESCRIPTION	WATER	CARBOHYDRATE
Easy runs lasting less than 1 hour	Optional but probably not worth the bother	None
Runs lasting 45 to 60 minutes and featuring substantial amounts of running in Zone 3 or higher	Optional	30 g per hour
Runs lasting 1 to 2 hours	Personal preference (whatever is most comfortable)	Take in 30 g per hour in roughly half of these runs; withhold carbs in the other half
Runs lasting longer than 2 hours	Drink by thirst	At least 30 g per hour
Race simulation runs	Drink by thirst	At least 60 g per hour or maximum tolerable amount

The integrated training-nutrition plans in Chapters 10 and 11 give you fueling recommendations that are consistent with these guidelines.

SPORTS DRINKS AND ENERGY GELS

In theory, you could get carbohydrates during your runs from whole fruit, pastries, or soft drinks. In practice, this wouldn't be a very good idea, and not only because that could be messy and unwieldy. Only specially formulated sports drinks and energy gels provide carbs in the optimal amounts and concentrations to maximize performance without extra ingredients (fat, fiber) that would slow the absorption of carbs and increase the risk of GI distress. Similarly, sports drinks and pure water are the only liquids that you should use while running.

While you probably know you should get your carbs from sports drinks and energy gels, you might be wondering about whether you should use one or the other or both. An energy gel is essentially a sports drink without water. Most sports drinks and energy gels contain the same types of carbohydrates and similar amounts of sodium and other minerals, which are included to replace some of the electrolytes that the body loses through perspiration during running. Because energy gels lack water, you should never rely on them exclusively to meet your nutrition needs when you run; you must also drink water to get a performance benefit matching that of sports drinks.

It is possible to combine the use of sports drinks and energy gels in workouts and races, but it can be tricky. Washing down an energy gel with a sports drink is tantamount to drinking a much more concentrated sports drink, and research has shown that solutions with carb concentrations above 12 percent are not absorbed or tolerated as well. Some runners can get away with it, whereas others can't. Too often runners find out the hard way—in races—that they can't. Rochelle Cuff did so in the 2011 Big D Marathon in Dallas. Midway through the race she drank a full cup of Powerade immediately after swallowing a packet of gel. Her digestive system reacted swiftly and badly to the sudden onslaught of carbs. She was forced to make three bathroom stops and, although she managed to finish the race, she missed her goal time by three minutes—about the same amount of time she spent in Porta Potties.

Using both a sports drink and energy gels in the same workout or race can be an effective way to take in more carbs than you could get from a sports drink alone, but it's usually safest to use them sequentially. For example, you might wash down a gel with water, wait fifteen minutes, then sip some sports drink, wait another fifteen minutes, then wash down another gel with water, and so forth.

Sports drinks and energy gels have different advantages and disadvantages. Sports drinks are more convenient than energy gels in the sense that they provide both carbohydrate and water from a single source. Energy gels are more convenient in the sense that they are more portable. If you have access to water from drinking fountains or other sources on your runs, you may choose to carry gels and stop periodically to drink instead of lugging a heavy bottle of sports drink.

Another advantage that energy gels have in relation to sports drinks is that gels allow you to adjust the balance of carbs and water that you consume to meet your particular needs. You can have a little gel with a lot of water if you want more fluid than carbs, or you can have a lot of gel with a little water if you want more carbs than fluid. By contrast, with sports drinks you're stuck with a fixed ratio of carbs and fluid.

Most sports drinks are 5 to 8 percent carbohydrate solutions. That's no accident. At this concentration the typical sports drink provides about the right amount of carbs and water to maximize performance in most exercise activities. But running is different from other exercise activities. The body cannot tolerate as much fluid intake during running because of the stomach jostling that it entails. Runners typically drink only 200 to 800 ml per hour during races. Cyclists, on the other hand, typically consume more than one full liter per hour in competition. Because the carbohydrate concentration in sports drinks is fixed, a runner who drinks a sports drink at a maximum tolerable rate of 200 to 800 ml per hour is not only getting less fluid than a cyclist who drinks more than 1000 ml per hour but is also getting less carbohydrate.

This wouldn't be such a bad thing if the body's capacity to absorb carbohydrate were also reduced during running compared to cycling and other activities. But in fact the maximum rate of carb absorption during running is the same as it is during cycling and other activities: between 60 and 90 g per hour. So, if you use a sports drink to fuel your workouts and races and you consume as much as you are comfortable drinking, you might not get as much carbohydrate as you could absorb and benefit from. But if you use energy gels and water as an alternative or as a supplement to the sports drink, you can get all the carbohydrate you can use without getting more fluid than you can tolerate.

Let's consider a specific example. Gatorade supplies 14 g of carbohydrate per 8-ounce serving. During a hard run you might be comfortable drinking 16 ounces (473 ml) of Gatorade per hour and no more. That would give you 28 g of carbs per hour, or slightly less than the 30 g of carbs per hour that is considered to be the minimum requirement for a measurable improvement in performance. A packet of Clif Shot energy gel provides 22 g of carbs. If you follow label directions and consume two packets per hour throughout a hard run, you'll take in 44 g of carbs per hour, easily meeting the minimum requirement for performance enhancement. By washing your Clif Shots down with 16 ounces of water per hour you may better meet your total nutrition needs without increased risk of GI distress.

CARBS IN RACES VS. CARBS IN WORKOUTS

As I suggested earlier in the chapter, falling short of the required rate of carbohydrate intake for maximum performance is not a big deal in most workouts. In races, however, you want to be sure to take in at least 60 g of carbs per hour or as much carbohydrate as you can comfortably tolerate. Unless you are able to tolerate significantly greater amounts of fluid than most runners, you will not be able to get all of the carbs you could use from a sports drink alone. You will need to supplement the sports drink with gels or rely on gels and water completely—unless, of course, you have trouble stomaching gels, as some runners do.

If you intend to use the official sports drink of your next marathon or half marathon during the race, it is important that you fuel at least some of your training runs with it for the sake of familiarization. If you happen to like this sports drink, you might as well use it throughout the training process. Otherwise, it's okay to use a product you prefer in all of your runs except your race-simulation workouts. While many marathons and half marathons have an energy gel sponsor as well as a sports drink sponsor, gels are typically available only at a single aid station along the course. So if you intend to rely on gels to any significant degree, you will have to carry them. The advantage here is that you can carry the product of your choice.

CHOOSING THE RIGHT DRINK AND GEL

There is a wide variety of sports drinks and energy gels on the market to choose from. While each brand claims to be more effective than the rest, there is little in the way of scientific comparisons of the various products. The most important factor to consider in choosing products to use in training is not the scientific claims you see in the advertisements for the various products but your body's response to them. It is likely that you will get the most benefit from the drink or gel that tastes best and sits most comfortably in your stomach for the simple reason that you will consume and absorb more of it than you would of a product that your taste buds or tummy rejected.

Not all products are deserving of road testing, however. I recommend that you avoid "low-calorie" and "low-sugar" sports drinks, such as Ultima Replenisher, that contain less than 10 g of carbohydrate per 12-ounce serving, unless you can't tolerate products with higher carbohydrate concentrations. Also avoid energy gels and sports drinks such as Gleukos that contain only one type of carbohydrate. The intestine absorbs different types of carbohydrates through separate channels. When a sports drink or energy gel contains more than one type of carbohydrate, the different types are able to enter the bloodstream simultaneously through separate channels instead of getting backed up at a single entryway as the carbs from single-carb drinks and gels do. Therefore your total carbohydrate absorption rate is faster with multi-carb products. Look for two or more of the following ingredients on the product label: brown rice syrup, dextrose, fructose, glucose, honey, maltodextrin, sucrose, and sugar.

Steer clear as well of sports drinks and energy gels that boast of providing "lasting energy" because they contain "complex carbs" instead of "simple sugars." While lasting energy sounds good, what you really need during intense exercise is *fast* energy, and any supplement that provides "lasting" energy provides it *slowly*. Even during easy workouts, your muscles burn carbohydrate at a much faster rate than you could ever replace it with carbs consumed in a sports drink. The only fuel source that needs to last during exercise is the carbohydrate stored as glycogen in your muscles and liver, because when these stores run low, you bonk. A sports drink that provides fast energy allows your muscles to conserve glycogen and thus extends endurance.

A sports drink or energy gel that is designed to provide lasting energy will deliver carbs too slowly to delay the glycogen bonk. Examples include products that contain large starches, which take forever to break down into usable glucose, and sports drinks whose main sugar is galactose, which must pass through the liver before it reaches the muscles and therefore delivers energy at half the rate other sugars do.

Some runners are concerned that consuming simple sugars during exercise will cause an "insulin spike" followed by a "blood-sugar crash" that causes fatigue. Although drinking a sports drink containing simple sugars at rest might indeed cause such a response, this "reactive hypoglycemia" phenomenon does not occur during exercise, when the body functions in a stress state in which the blood sugar level is tightly controlled regardless of what sort of nutrition is consumed. Also, insulin spikes and blood sugar crashes tend to follow a large, single dose of sugar, whereas runners consume small amounts of sugar at frequent intervals.

As I suggested earlier, electrolyte minerals—namely sodium, chloride, potassium, and magnesium—are useful ingredients in sports drinks and energy gels because they replace a portion of the minerals lost in sweat. Whereas electrolytes have been falsely credited for enhancing rehydration and preventing muscle cramps, their greatest real benefit may be that they stimulate thirst and increased drinking. Some low-calorie sports drinks and fitness waters contain very low levels of electrolytes. I recommend that you choose a sports drink containing enough electrolytes that you can actually taste them.

A few sports drinks and gels contain a small amount of protein, which may reduce muscle damage during runs. I'll have more to say on this topic in Chapter 8. A number of energy gels contain caffeine.

I will address the subject of caffeine as a performance enhancer in Chapter 6.

There is no known benefit associated with any sports drink ingredient besides those I have already named. Many products include fancy extras such as "lactate buffers" and antioxidants that have no effect on endurance performance in any amount and are often included in amounts too small for the body to even register. In my view such extras can only get in the way of the ingredients that really do work. A good sports drink or energy gel's list of ingredients is short—twelve to fifteen constituents.

DEVELOPING A RACE NUTRITION PLAN

As I suggested earlier in the chapter, the point of fueling your body during training runs is not only to enhance your performance in those workouts but also to give you an opportunity to develop and practice a fueling plan for your next event. It is not necessary to fuel every workout as though it were a race or to use every workout as race-nutrition practice. It is enough to set aside two or three of your longest runs or your longer runs at race intensity in which to use the same product or products you will use during your race and at the same rate you hope to use them in competition.

There are several factors to consider when developing a personal race nutrition plan. These factors include the distance of the race (many runners require different plans for marathons and half marathons), your individual tolerance for fluid and carbohydrate intake while running, and your preference for sports drinks or gels as a primary carbohydrate source. Runners who weigh each factor against their personal experience typically find that one of five basic race nutrition plans works best for them. In Chapter 7 I will describe these five plans and explain how to choose the one that's best for you.

Use your long training runs and your race-pace training sessions to develop (or choose) a race nutrition plan. Once you have settled on a provisional plan, use your hardest, most race-specific workout before a marathon or half marathon to test that plan. In the marathon training plans presented in Chapter 11, this workout is called the Simulator.

The Simulator was developed by brothers Keith and Kevin Hanson, co–head coaches of the Hansons-Brooks Distance Project, a team of elite runners based in Rochester, Michigan. As the name suggests, the workout's purpose is to simulate an upcoming marathon race as closely as possible without stressing you to the point of ruining the flow of your training. It is intended to put the finishing touches on your marathon-specific fitness and demonstrate your ability to achieve a time/pace goal for the marathon. (For info on half marathons, see the end of the chapter.)

The format couldn't be simpler. The Simulator consists of 26.2 km (roughly 16.3 miles) of running at one's goal marathon pace. Why 26.2 km? Two reasons. First, at 62 percent of the full marathon distance, 16.3 miles is long enough to challenge and increase your capacity to sustain a targeted marathon pace and to provide a legitimate indication of how realistic your marathon goal is. Yet it's not so long that it will destroy your legs for the next three days and thereby disrupt the flow of training.

The second rationale for the 26.2 km distance is purely psychological. The difference between running, say, a 16-mile marathon-pace run and a 26.2 km Simulator is almost entirely symbolic, but the symbolism is important. Consciously approaching the Simulator as a "metric marathon" enhances your awareness of the workout as proof of your readiness to run 26.2 miles at a desired pace a few weeks later. It makes the workout just a bit more confidence-boosting than a virtually identical workout lacking that layer of symbolism.

In marathon training it's vitally important to arrive at the start line feeling confident in your ability to achieve your goal. Such confidence comes from having proven your readiness in training. The less of a reach your race goal seems from your recent achievements in training, the more confident you will be, and the more confident you are, the more likely it is that you will achieve your goal. It's nice to be able to stand on that starting line and think, *Yeah, I'm nervous, but I've already run the pace I want to run today for 26.2 km. . . .*

The Hansons usually have their runners perform the Simulator five weeks before a marathon. That works for elite runners who run such high mileage that they need three full weeks to taper for their race, but for us mortals it's better to run the Simulator closer to race day—between four and two weeks out. Again, the idea is to put the finishing touches on your marathon fitness, so it needs to be one of the last hard workouts you do.

Before you start the Simulator you'll want to do the same warm-up you intend to do before your marathon. I recommend a mile of jogging, a few mobility exercises (such as giant walking lunges), and a few strides (20-second runs at 5K race pace). Try to do the workout on a course that's very similar to the course of your upcoming marathon. When it came time for the Hansons team to run the Simulator ahead of the 2008 men's Olympic trials marathon, held in New York City, they took a nine-hour bus trip from eastern Michigan to the Big Apple and ran it in Central Park.

Treat the Simulator as a full dress rehearsal for your marathon. In addition to running it on the actual racecourse or a similar route, do it at the same time of day as your marathon, wear the same clothes and shoes you will wear in the race, and, of course, practice your race nutrition plan. If you plan to rely on the official marathon sports drink to any extent, use that brand and flavor in the Simulator. If you plan to use both the official sports drink and water, give yourself access to both. And if you plan to carry energy gels during the race, then carry the same brand and flavor in the Simulator.

Before you start the Simulator, visit your event's website, call up the course map, and find the exact locations of the fluid stations. When you run the Simulator, drink at distance points that match the locations of the marathon fluid stations. For example, if the first three fluid stations are located at 1.1, 2.2, and 3.3 miles, then drink at 1.1, 2.2, and 3.3 miles of the Simulator. If possible, recruit a friend or family member to accompany you on a bike and hand you the bottle at the appropriate distances. If you must carry your own fluid, resist any temptation to drink between "aid stations" and be aware that the extra weight is likely to add a few seconds per mile to your pace.

If all goes well, use the same nutrition plan you tested in the Simulator in your race. If you encounter a problem, look over all five race nutrition plans again and choose the most sensible alternative. For example, if you choose a plan that entails use of energy gels and you discover that you have trouble getting them down when running at your marathon pace (which is not unheard of), then switch to a plan that excludes gel use.

Since pacing is a critical element of this workout, you need to be able to monitor your pace throughout it. One option is to run on a marked course or on a route with known mile landmarks, wear a stopwatch, and check your splits as you pass the markers or landmarks. A second option is to wear a speed and distance device such as a Garmin Forerunner. A third option is to have your fluid support cyclist use a bike with a cyclometer that measures time, distance covered, and average speed.

The Hansons don't prescribe a formal half-marathon Simulator, but the toughest and most race-specific workouts they have their runners do in half-marathon training are very close to being half of the marathon Simulator, or 13.1 km (8.1 miles) at goal race pace. The half-marathon training plans in Chapter 10 prescribe half-marathon Simulators, which you should approach in precisely the same way you do marathon Simulators.

BEFORE YOU HIT THE SHOWER

The first thing you should do after completing a Simulator or any challenging run is take in some recovery nutrition. Consuming the right nutrients—namely, carbohydrate, protein, water, and antioxidants—within forty-five minutes of finishing up a hard run will accelerate your recovery and enable you to perform better in the next run. I'll present complete guidelines for recovery nutrition in Chapter 8.

THE TAPER DIET

The final weeks of training before an important race such as a marathon or half marathon are commonly referred to as a taper period. The term originated not in running but in swimming, coined in the 1950s by the legendary Australian coach Forbes Carlile, who noticed that his athletes tended to race better after their training had been briefly curtailed, whether by accident or by design. Carlile thereafter "tapered down" the training of his swimmers intentionally before major competitions.

Tapering is now practiced universally in all endurance sports and in many other fitness-based sports, from powerlifting to track and field. Distance runners benefit as much as athletes in any other sport from the practice of reducing the training load before races. A sharp taper in the final weeks before a marathon or half marathon allows your body to fully absorb and recover from previous hard training and triggers other favorable physiological changes that enable you to race at the highest level.

The taper period is not all about training, however. In fact, the changes you make in your diet at this time should be just as significant as those you make in your workouts and could have an equally beneficial effect on your race performance. Training-nutrition synergy is important throughout the process of preparing for a marathon or half marathon, but during the taper period the interplay between workouts and food demands even more careful attention. If you execute both components of the taper correctly you will be a much stronger runner on race morning than you were just a couple of weeks before.

MORE THAN RESTING UP

Tapering is so familiar today that most runners probably assume it has always been done, but it hasn't. Although it now seems self-evident that resting up after a period of hard training enhances subsequent race performance, this particular pattern of cause and effect was largely invisible to athletes before the middle of the last century. "People thought [that] to keep condition you had to train pretty hard right up to the event," said Forbes Carlile regarding the prevailing attitude among his fellow swim coaches prior to his introduction of tapering to the sport.

The same attitude prevailed in running until the great Czech runner Emil Zátopek stumbled upon the same insight that struck Carlile at almost the same time on another continent and in a different sport. While training for the 1950 European Games Zátopek fell seriously ill and was hospitalized for two weeks, during which time he was unable to run a single step. Released from the hospital just two days before the Games, Zátopek won the 10,000 meters by a full lap and then won the 5,000 meters by twenty-three seconds. Throughout the rest of his career Zátopek made sure to rest up (outside the hospital!) before racing.

Winner of three gold medals in the 1952 Olympics, Zátopek was recognized as the greatest runner of his day and so his methods—including tapering—became broadly emulated by other runners. New Zealand running coach Arthur Lydiard incorporated tapering into the four-phase training system he developed in the late 1950s, which became an almost universal paradigm for the training of middle- and long-distance runners. (I'll say more about Lydiard's system in Chapter 9.)

Exercise scientists began to study the effects of various tapering protocols on swimming performance in the 1960s. Soon they expanded their investigations to include cyclists and runners. The taper became a popular object of scientific inquiry because it is an inherently short-term phenomenon and therefore much easier to control and manipulate than other aspects of the training process. Exercise scientists continue to study tapering methods intensively today.

There are two basic scientific approaches to the subject of tapering. Some studies aim to identify and quantify the performance-enhancing physiological adaptations that occur in response to a short-term reduction in training volume. These adaptations are now known to include increases in muscle glycogen storage, blood volume, and neuromuscular power. Other studies have compared the effects of different tapering protocols on performance. The main variables are the duration of the taper, the degree of initial training reduction, the rate of training reduction throughout the taper, and the amount of high-intensity training that is performed during the taper. It's impossible to draw uniform, universally applicable conclusions from the total body of such studies, but there have been some consistent findings that provide useful, general guidelines for tapering.

TAPER TRAINING GUIDELINES

The best results seem to follow when the taper is at least one week long, the volume reduction is at least 50 percent compared to the previous week, and the tapering period includes a fair amount of race-pace efforts (instead of being entirely low intensity). For example, in a study from East Carolina University, a group of runners lopped an average of twenty-nine seconds off their 5K race times after completing an eight-day taper in which their training volume was reduced by 70 percent compared to the previous week and a small number of race-pace intervals were run each day.

As a general rule, the higher your peak training volume is, the longer your prerace taper should be. Indeed, one of the reasons that runners before Emil Zátopek did not taper is that they tended to train very lightly compared to today's standards—so lightly that they didn't really need to taper. If your last heavy week of training includes 20 to 40 miles of running (or the equivalent in running and cross-training combined), then a one-week taper is sufficient. If your peak training week includes 41 to 80 miles or the equivalent, then a two-week taper is necessary. And if your last hard week includes more than 80 miles of running or the equivalent, then you should taper for three full weeks, as most elite runners do before marathons and half marathons. The training plans presented in Chapters 10 and 11 follow these guidelines.

Note that it's not the distance of your race—marathon or half marathon—that should determine the length of your taper but the amount of training you do. If you run 41 to 80 miles per week in training, for example, you should do a two-week taper regardless of whether you're preparing for a marathon or a half marathon. As we'll see later, most of the nutritional guidelines for the taper period apply to both marathons and half marathons.

The most common mistake that runners make in tapering is doing too little high-intensity training during the final one to three weeks before racing. Research has consistently shown that a taper featuring a fair amount of high-intensity training is more effective than one featuring only easy efforts. While the overall volume of high-intensity running you do during the taper period should be reduced compared to the peak training period, your easy training should be reduced to a much greater degree.

Most of the high-intensity training efforts you do during the taper period should be undertaken at your goal race pace or slightly faster. You want your body and mind to be as fully adapted to this specific intensity level as possible. You may also do a very small amount of near-maximal intensity running for a last-minute boost in power and economy.

Whether you're training for a full or half marathon, I recommend that you perform your last "hard" workout three days before your race. This workout should feature enough high-intensity work to leave you mildly fatigued. Your final two days of training should consist of nothing more than warm-ups and maybe a few relaxed sprints to keep the nervous system primed.

NUTRITION DURING THE TAPER PERIOD

The taper diet that I recommend to runners who are preparing to race a marathon or half marathon has four steps: (1) reducing calorie intake, (2) fat loading, (3) caffeine fasting, and (4) carb loading.

Let's take a closer look at each of these steps.

STEP ONE: REDUCING CALORIE INTAKE

The purpose of this step is to prevent weight gain during the taper. Naturally, your "calorie taper" should start whenever your training taper does, so if you do a one-week taper, you would also start to eat less a week from race day.

Weight gain within a prerace taper period is quite common. A week before the 2009 Boston Marathon Liz Plosser, a magazine editor in Chicago, stepped onto the scale and freaked out. She had gained a couple of pounds in the few days since she had started her taper. Liz hastily entered the phrase "marathon taper weight gain" into a Google search box and—to her great relief—found an article written by an expert who explained that since muscle glycogen stores increase substantially during a prerace taper, and because glycogen is stored with water, which is heavy, a certain amount of weight gain is normal and even desirable in the last week or so before a race.

That's true enough, but fat gain is also common during the taper period, and it is most certainly *not* beneficial. The problem is that runners do not start to eat less automatically as soon as they cut back on their training to rest up for a marathon or half marathon. It takes a little time for the appetite to adjust to the new, lower rate of daily energy expenditure. On top of that, there's the force of habit: Runners get used to eating a lot at the height of their training for a big race. For these reasons, unless you make a conscious effort to eat less during your taper, you will probably continue to eat as much as you did at the height of your training and consequently gain harmful fat weight as well as harmless water weight.

No runner gains more than 3 or 4 pounds during a taper, but even the small amount of fat accumulation that can easily occur might turn a new PR into an agonizing near miss. Consider Julie, a hypothetical runner who runs 50 miles in her peak training week, 30 miles in the first week of a two-week taper, and 15 miles in the first six days of race week. Assuming an average net burn rate of 82 calories per mile (net calorie burn is the number of calories burned during running minus the number of calories the runner would have burned had she sat around instead), Julie burns roughly 3,900 fewer calories during her thirteen days of tapering than she burned during her last thirteen days of peak-level training. If she continues eating as she did at the height of her training, Julie will accumulate an energy surplus of 3,900 calories during her taper. In principle, every 3,500 calories of surplus eating results in 1 pound of weight gain. So Julie will gain more than a pound of body fat in the last two weeks before her race if she doesn't eat less. If Julie is a four-hour marathoner, that extra pound will add about a minute and a half to her finish time.

To prevent taper-period weight gain you need to reduce your daily calorie intake by an amount that equals the reduction in daily calorie burning that comes with running less. To attain this balance you must reduce your daily calorie intake by 0.63 multiplied by your weight in pounds for each mile that is eliminated from your training load during the taper period. To return to our hypothetical example, Julie ran 7.14 miles per day during her last week of hard training and only 4.28 miles per day during the first week of her taper. That's a decrease of 2.86 miles per day. Assuming she weighs 130 pounds, Julie needs to reduce her eating by 234 calories per day in that first taper week to prevent weight gain. And in the first six days of race week, when she runs just 2.5 miles a day, she'll need to cut back by another 146 calories per day.

If reduced calorie intake were the only dietary change you made in the taper period you could easily achieve the necessary reduction by subtracting the right number of calories from your normal meals and/or snacks. But because you're making other changes as well (namely, fat loading followed by carbo loading), it's easier to calculate the number of calories you need to consume to maintain your current weight—

given your reduced training volume—and then aim to consume that number of calories through the foods that make up your taper diet.

Online tools make these calculations fairly easy. My personal favorite can be found here: nutritiondata.self.com/tools/calories-burned. Plug in your age, gender, height, weight, and lifestyle, plus your daily amounts and intensities of exercise during the taper period, and you'll get a fairly accurate estimate of the number of calories you need to consume each day to maintain a stable weight.

STEP TWO: FAT LOADING

In Chapter 1, you will recall, I advised you not to maintain a high-fat diet as your normal training diet because although a high-fat diet increases fat-burning capacity, it also deprives the body of the carbohydrate needed to handle a heavy training load. But a brief fat-loading phase that begins within two weeks of an upcoming event allows you to increase your fat-burning capacity for a race without compromising your training. Fat-loading is not a mandatory step of the taper diet and can be skipped if you are not comfortable with even a short period of high-fat eating.

In 2001 Vicki Lambert, an exercise scientist at the University of Cape Town, South Africa, examined the effects of a ten-day high-fat diet followed by three days of carbohydrate loading on the fat-burning capacity and performance of trained cyclists. Her hypothesis was that fat loading would increase reliance on fat and decrease reliance on glycogen as exercise fuel, while subsequent carbo loading would maximize glycogen stores without negating the effect of fat loading. With more glycogen available and less glycogen being used, the cyclists would be less likely to hit the wall and their performance would improve.

It worked. Lambert observed that the cyclists burned significantly more fat and less carbohydrate during a long time trial when it was preceded by fat loading and carbo loading than when it was preceded by carbo loading alone. Most noteworthy, the high-fat/carbo-loading treatment was also associated with improved performance. On average, the cyclists completed the 20 km time trial 4.5 percent faster after the high-fat/carbo-loading diet.

Follow-up studies with somewhat different designs have confirmed the metabolic findings of this study but have not duplicated its performance benefit. No one has yet investigated the effect of fat loading before carbo-loading on marathon performance. My hunch is that such an investigation would find that it works for at least some runners because runners are more likely to hit the wall in a marathon than trained cyclists are to hit the wall in a 20 km cycling time trial preceded by two hours of moderate-intensity cycling.

Indeed, the benefits of fat loading followed by carbo loading on marathon performance seemed likely enough to me when I read Lambert's study that I decided to try it out for myself. I first conducted a trial run before a low-key half marathon, fat loading for three days and then carbo loading for one day. I knew this highly condensed version of the method wouldn't give me the full effect, but it would give me a sense of how my body (and mind) would react to an unusually high level of fat intake. A word of caution here: No runner should ever experiment with such a drastic departure from his or her normal diet for the first time before an important race. Follow my example by trying out fat loading for three days before a lower-priority race, prior to doing it for real before an important marathon or half marathon. If it doesn't go well you will at least be glad you didn't fat load for the first time with sixteen or twenty weeks of hard training and dreams of a new PR at stake.

My own test went fine, so I engaged in a full ten-day fat load followed by three days of carbo loading prior to my next marathon. It was not exactly a controlled experiment, as I did some other things differently than I had in preparing for past marathons, but I had a great race and I believe that the fat loading had something to do with it. So I'm comfortable recommending it to you.

There is nothing at all unhealthy about getting 65 percent of your daily calories from fat for ten days, especially if you rely on the foods I recommend on page 104, so don't let that concern you. Getting two-thirds of your calories from fat is not easy, though. It requires that virtually everything you eat be high in fat. Switching to such a diet from the typical carb-rich runner's diet is rather disruptive, and because the list of high-quality high-fat foods is quite short, it begins to feel monotonous very quickly. Within three days of starting my ten-day fat load I couldn't wait to get the damn thing over with.

It is impossible to increase fat consumption to 65 percent of total calories without simultaneously reducing carbohydrate intake, which causes feelings of heaviness and lethargy both during and between runs. Because fat loading begins immediately after the last hard week of training has been put in the books, however, its effect on performance is inconsequential. The deep malaise of carbohydrate deprivation could damage your psyche nevertheless, since you may feel as though half of your fitness has disappeared suddenly with a big race just around the corner. But I have found that the sluggish feeling associated with fat loading has the opposite impact on my mental state. During my fat-loading periods I look forward to the abrupt return to vitality I will enjoy when I switch to carbo loading. The combination of taper training and carbo loading always makes a runner feel ready to race, but in my experience the carbo-loaded state feels twice as energizing—almost superhuman—after fat loading.

Some caveats: The probable benefit of fat loading before a race is small enough that the practice may not be worthwhile for every runner. First of all, if your next important race is a half marathon and you anticipate completing it in less than two hours, you need not bother fat loading. It won't help you. Also, if your three-day fat-loading test does not go well, then you ought to skip step two of the taper diet without fearing that doing so will limit your performance significantly. And again, if you just don't like the idea of eating that much fat, go ahead and skip step two.

Alternatively, try a condensed, five-day fat-loading period followed by a single day of carbo loading. One study found that this protocol increased fat burning at race intensity about as much as a ten-day fat-loading period followed by three days of carbo loading, although it did not enhance performance in a 20 km cycling time trial preceded by two hours of moderate-intensity pedaling.

Given that this five-day alternative fat-loading period is half as long as the standard ten-day fat-loading period, you might assume that ten-day fat-loading periods are appropriate for marathons and five-day fat-loading periods are appropriate for half marathons. This is not necessarily the case. It's better to allow the duration of your fat-loading period to be determined by the length of your taper, which, remember, is in turn determined by your weekly running mileage, not by the length of your race.

If you train at low volumes and consequently taper just one week before races, then a five-day fat load should be your first option. The last thing you'll want to do when performing some of your toughest peak workouts in the second-to-last week before a race is deprive your body of the carbs it needs to complete these workouts successfully. If you run more and will thus taper for two or three weeks, then a ten-day fat load should be your first choice.

As I mentioned, there are not many high-quality foods that get more than 60 percent of their calories from fat. Those that do include avocados (83 percent), cheese (73 percent), Greek yogurt (63 percent), nuts (cashews, for example, are 73 percent fat), and olives (77 percent). With careful planning you can supplement these foods with others that contain slightly less fat—such as whole milk (49 percent), salmon (54 percent), and sardines (48 percent)—and still end up getting 65 percent of your day's total calories from fat.

It is not easy to maintain diet quality balance during a fat-loading period. In fact, you need not bother tracking your diet quality balance while fat loading. This period should not, however, be treated as a time when "anything goes." While plenty of fatty meats get more than 60 percent of their calories from fat (for example, bologna is 72 percent fat), I discourage you from eating them more than sparingly even when fat loading. Nor is it necessary to eliminate fruits and vegetables from your diet to get 65 percent of your daily calories from fat. A Caesar salad, for example, is 66 percent fat, thanks to the olive oil–based dressing.

If few high-quality foods are more than 65 percent fat, still fewer plant foods are so fat rich. Vegans and strict vegetarians who do not eat meat, fish, eggs, and dairy products should not attempt to fat load unless they are prepared to live on nothing but avocados, nuts, olives, and nondairy cheese for five or ten days.

To determine the percentage of a food's calories that come from fat, first find the number of fat grams per serving on the product label or on calorieking.com, then multiply this number by 9 (the number of calories in a gram of fat), and finally divide the result by the total number of calories per serving. For example, according to calorieking .com, pumpkin seeds contain 16 g of fat per ¼-cup serving. The number of fat calories in a serving of pumpkins seeds therefore is (16 g × 9 cal/g =) 144. The total number of calories in ¼-cup of pumpkin seeds is 200. So pumpkin seeds are (144 ÷ 200 =) 72 percent fat.

Table 5.1 presents a sample one-day fat-loading meal plan.

STEP THREE: CAFFEINE FASTING

This step begins either one or two weeks before race day (therefore it partially overlaps with the fat-loading phase) and continues until race morning. A caffeine fast is necessary to maximize the benefits of taking caffeine immediately before a race. If you do not normally consume caffeine or you do not plan to take caffeine before a race, this step can be skipped as well.

Like the other nutritional steps of the fat-loading period, the caffeine fast pertains to both marathons and half marathons. In fact, you'd be well advised to do a caffeine fast ahead of pre-competition caffeine use even if your race was a 100-meter sprint.

Caffeine is very similar in chemical structure to a compound called adenosine that the body produces naturally. Adenosine serves various

TABLE 5.1 *SAMPLE ONE-DAY FAT-LOADING MEAL PLAN*

MEAL	TOTAL CALORIES	FAT CALORIES
3-egg omelet with feta cheese and avocado	407	277
1.5 ounces dry-roasted cashews	244	178
Cream of chicken soup Caesar salad	500	314
Eden Foods All Mixed Up	160	110
6 ounces broiled salmon with lemon butter sauce Broccoli with Cheddar cheese sauce	592	360
Greek yogurt with fresh blueberries	256	153
TOTALS	2,159	1,392
PERCENTAGE OF DAY'S TOTAL CALORIES FROM FAT	65	

biological functions. In the brain it acts as a neurotransmitter—a chemical messenger that transmits signals from one brain cell to another. Many brain cells contain special adenosine receptors that adenosine molecules fit into like a key in a lock. When the brain is not releasing a lot of adenosine, the majority of adenosine receptors stand empty, and when the majority of adenosine receptors stand empty, a person feels wakeful and alert and signals travel quickly both within the brain and from the brain to the muscles. When the brain releases a lot of adenosine, which it does at nighttime, a person becomes sleepy and the brain slows down.

When caffeine is consumed, the drug (and it is a drug) crosses the blood-brain barrier and attaches itself to adenosine receptors, which can't tell the difference between caffeine and adenosine. With adenosine receptors thus occupied, adenosine is prevented from completing its mission of transmitting signals that induce drowsiness and slow down the brain. The perceived effects of caffeine's adenosine blockade—feelings of alertness, mental acuity, and physical energy—are familiar to every coffee drinker. But athletes know an additional set of effects. During exercise caffeine accelerates the transmission of signals from the brain to the muscles, reduces perceived effort, and enhances athletic performance.

Habitual caffeine use such as drinking coffee every day causes the brain to "upregulate" its adenosine receptors. This adaptation makes the brain more sensitive to the action of adenosine so that fewer adenosine molecules must attach themselves to receptors to cause sleepiness and brain slowing. Habituation also makes the brain less sensitive to the actions of caffeine. For runners, caffeine habituation has the important implication that it reduces the drug's benefit of performance enhancement.

In 2002 Canadian researchers compared the effects of preexercise caffeine intake on exercise performance in thirteen habitual caffeine users and eight nonusers. All twenty-one subjects ingested a fairly large dose of caffeine. An hour later they were required to pedal stationary bikes to exhaustion at a fixed high intensity. Two hours later they completed a second such ride, and three hours after that they did one more. This entire protocol was repeated on a separate occasion with the subjects receiving a placebo instead of caffeine. Habitual caffeine users were able to pedal 17.6 percent longer one hour after taking caffeine than they were an hour after receiving the placebo. But the nonusers got twice the benefit, and the discrepancy between caffeine's effects on habitual users and nonusers was even greater in the second and third rides undertaken three hours and six hours after caffeine ingestion.

The hard lesson of this study for coffee-loving runners is that, to get the maximum possible benefit from caffeine in a marathon or half marathon, one must be a nonuser or become one before the race. Many runners who normally drink coffee put this lesson into effect by engaging in what has become a traditional one-week caffeine fast before important races.

Whether a one-week fast is long enough to increase the performance-enhancing effect of preexercise caffeine use to the same level that nonusers enjoy is unknown. A 1998 study found that two- and four-day caffeine fasts made no difference. However, a study involving mice habituated to very high levels of caffeine intake showed that adenosine receptors were fully downregulated to normal levels after eight days of caffeine withdrawal, suggesting that eight days is long enough to reverse the effects of habituation.

While science has yet to determine whether the runner's traditional one-week prerace caffeine fast is sufficient, I am already certain that it works for me because I feel exceptionally energetic when I take caffeine before a race after a one-week fast, whereas caffeine's effect on my daily training runs is barely noticeable. My confidence in the effectiveness of a one-week caffeine fast is further bolstered by an incident that occurred three or four days into a fast that I did before the 2008 Silicon Valley Marathon. After eating my lunch on that day I suddenly noticed that I felt wired and euphoric, as though I had just drunk an extra-large mug of extra-strong coffee. Then I realized that the tiny piece of dark chocolate I'd just eaten as a postlunch treat contained a little caffeine, and my sensitivity to caffeine's effects was apparently so heightened already that this tiny amount altered my state of mind more than the larger amounts of caffeine I was accustomed to.

In addition to giving me confidence that a seven-day caffeine fast is enough to significantly boost the effect of prerace caffeine use for me, this incident reminded me that it's important to eliminate *all* sources of caffeine from the diet during race week. Be vigilant when doing your own caffeine fasts.

The more caffeine you normally ingest, the longer you'll need to fast to get something close to a nonuser's level of benefit from prerace caffeine use. Of course, the more caffeine you normally ingest, the harder this is likely to be. Caffeine withdrawal can be very unpleasant for the person who normally drinks several cups of coffee (or several energy drinks or whatever) per day. Common symptoms include headache, sleepiness, irritability, and sluggish thinking. I normally drink one big mug of strong coffee per day and consume no other caffeinated beverages. If you use caffeine in similar amounts, then the one-week caffeine fast that works for me will probably work for you. If you normally drink a lot of coffee or other caffeinated beverages and you can bear a ten-day or two-week caffeine fast before your most important events, then go for it. Otherwise, trust that a week's withdrawal is worthwhile.

The practice of using caffeine to enhance race performance after a caffeine fast does not work well for every runner, so it's a good idea to practice it in training first. Irit Levy wishes she had. Normally a heavy caffeine user (five or six cups of coffee a day), Levy decided to take herself off coffee for two months before running the 2009 Sydney Morning Herald Half Marathon. She then used caffeinated energy gels during the race. Expecting a physical boost, she got a mental blow instead. The caffeine went straight to her head, causing her to feel dizzy and wobbly. Needless to say, the race did not turn out well for her, and she hasn't used caffeine in a race since that day. To avoid such a surprise, experiment with a one-week fast followed by prerun or in-run caffeine use before running a Simulator workout or a low-priority race, and repeat the process before an important race only if this test goes well.

STEP FOUR: CARBOHYDRATE LOADING

The fourth and final step of the taper diet is the one that most runners are familiar with: carbohydrate loading. Various carbo-loading proto-

cols have come and gone over the years. I recommend three days of
eating 70 percent carbohydrate after a ten-day fat load and one day
of eating 10 g per kilogram of body weight after a five-day fat load.
Runners who skip fat loading are free to choose either of these carbo-
loading protocols.

The original carbohydrate loading method was an extreme two-
phase protocol developed by a Swedish physiologist named Gunvar
Ahlborg in the 1960s. The first phase was actually a glycogen *depletion*
phase that began one week before a big race with a long workout that
served to severely reduce glycogen stores in the muscles. What remained of these stores was then finished off with four days of low-carb
dieting. And when I say "low" I mean very low: just 10 percent of total
calories. Phase two of Ahlborg's protocol consisted of three days of
extremely high-carb eating. And when I say "high" I mean very high:
90 percent of total calories.

The idea behind phase one was that depleting the muscles of their
glycogen stores would trigger a sort of biochemical panic response that
would vastly increase the muscles' capacity to store glycogen when
carbohydrate was reintroduced into the diet. Ahlborg referred to this
phenomenon as glycogen supercompensation.

Later research demonstrated that such depletion was unnecessary.
Athletes could increase their muscle glycogen stores just as much by
simply tapering down their training so that they did not use as much
glycogen and then increasing their carb intake during the final one
to three days before racing. This discovery came as welcome news to
athletes who had suffered through Ahlborg's original protocol. Severe
glycogen depletion is extremely unpleasant, causing irritability, mental
confusion, and lethargy; and training in such a state is even more unpleasant. While tapering for the 1976 Olympic Marathon Frank
Shorter felt so miserable during a run on his second day of carb avoid-
ance that he snapped, gorging on M&M's and beer as soon as he returned home.

Within the past decade most serious runners have transitioned
from the Ahlborg protocol to carbo loading without prior glycogen depletion. Nowadays even meticulous elite-level marathoners may do
nothing more complicated or drastic than increasing their carbohydrate

intake to 70 percent of total calories for the last three days before racing. With the advent of fat loading, however, we're seeing growing numbers of runners do something that looks a lot more like the old two-phase method of carbo loading.

There are some crucial differences between fat loading and glycogen depletion, though. While fat loading does reduce muscle glycogen stores, this reduction is not the purpose of fat loading. That is why fat loading does not require that runners perform an exhaustive workout one week before a race or reduce their carbohydrate intake to 10 percent of total calories. Consequently, glycogen levels drop much less with fat loading than with glycogen depletion and the symptoms of lethargy and mental cloudiness are much milder.

The same approach to carbo loading that works best without prior fat loading works best with it as well. If you do a ten-day fat-loading phase that starts two weeks before your race, switch to carbo loading for the final three days before your event (plus breakfast on race morning). Getting 70 percent of your total calories from carbohydrate during this period will suffice to maximize your muscle glycogen stores. If you do a five-day fat-loading phase that begins six days before your race, switch to carbo loading for the last day before your event (plus breakfast on race morning). In this case you'll want to really crank up your carbohydrate intake on that one day—aiming for 10 g per kilogram of body weight—to guarantee that your muscles' glycogen storage capacity is fully saturated.

It's okay to use supplements and processed foods you don't normally eat to meet your carbohydrate needs during this brief loading period. You'll find it easier to get 10 g of carbs per kilogram you weigh with the aid of recovery drinks such as Endurox R[4] or even adult nutrition shakes such as Boost and Ensure.

Tables 5.2 and 5.3 present sample one-day carbo-loading meal plans. The first plan supplies carbs in the amount of 70 percent of total calories and the second provides 10 g of carbohydrate per kilogram of body weight for a hypothetical runner weighing 70 kg. Few runners consume such large amounts of carbohydrate even when they think they're carbo loading, and they pay a price for it in races. This was shown in a study conducted by Trent Stellingwerff of the Canadian Sports Centre in

TABLE 5.2 *SAMPLE ONE-DAY CARBO-LOADING MEAL PLAN: 70 PERCENT OF TOTAL CALORIES*

This meal plan is appropriate for runners aiming to get 70 percent of their calories from carbs for three days. Note that the day's 2,149-calorie total is suitable only for runners who are burning 2,149 calories per day during the final three days before a race. Be sure to scale your carbo-loading diet so that your total daily calorie intake equals your total daily caloric expenditure and you avoid last-minute weight gain.

MEAL	TOTAL CALORIES	CARBOHYDRATE CALORIES
Oatmeal with raisins and almond slivers Smoothie with orange juice, banana, spinach, and strawberries	564	432
Carrot sticks with ranch dip	70	20
Split Pea Soup (page 62) Toasted whole wheat bread with peanut butter V8 Juice	457	267
Endurox R^4 Recovery Drink (postrun)	270	208
Whole wheat spaghetti with tomato sauce Garden salad with vinaigrette dressing	688	498
Apple	100	96
TOTALS	2,149	1,521
PERCENTAGE OF DAY'S TOTAL CALORIES FROM CARBOHYDRATE	70.7	

Victoria. Stellingwerff tracked the diets of 257 runners during the final five weeks before the 2009 London Marathon. Only thirty-one of these runners managed to consume even 7 g of carbs per kilogram of body weight on the eve of the race. Those thirty-one runners were duly rewarded, completing the marathon on average 13.4 percent faster than did a group of runners matched for gender, age, body weight, training volume, and marathon experience. Most of this difference came in the final 4.5 miles, where the runners who had eaten fewer carbs the day before hit the wall and slowed down precipitously and the runners who had carbo loaded properly slowed down much less.

Carbo loading does not aid performance in events lasting less than two hours. So if your next race is a half marathon and you are a sub-two-hour performer, you can eat normally during race week. But when you do carbo load, do it right—unlike 226 of the 257 London Marathon participants involved in the study I just described!

TABLE 5.3 *SAMPLE ONE-DAY CARBO-LOADING MEAL PLAN: 10 G/KG OF BODY WEIGHT*

This meal plan is appropriate for a runner weighing 70 kilograms (154 pounds) who is aiming to consume 10 grams of carbs per kilogram of body weight for one day. To reach this target the runner will need to consume 2,800 calories of carbs, which is a far greater number of calories than a 70 kg runner would ever burn the day before running a marathon, but that's okay—it's just one day. To avoid extravagantly overeating in such circumstances, however, it's best to get as few calories as possible from anything other than carbohydrate.

I've deliberately left total calories off this table to underscore the point that they are not relevant in a one-day carbo load. Nor do carbohydrate calories matter, per se, or carbs as a percentage of total calories. Stay focused on the absolute amount of carbs you're taking in—that is, grams.

MEAL	CARBOHYDRATE GRAMS
Blueberry pancakes (four 6-inch) with maple syrup Tall glass of orange juice	201
Large banana Ensure brand adult nutrition shake	81
Ramen noodle soup, double serving Plain bagel with 100% fruit spread Cherry juice	179
Large banana Ensure brand adult nutrition shake	81
Stir-fried vegetables with 1½ cups of brown rice	93
Large banana Ensure brand adult nutrition shake	81
TOTAL CARBOHYDRATE GRAMS	716

ALMOST THERE

It is often said that getting to the starting line of a marathon or half marathon is half the battle. This is true. There are lots of ways for both the training and nutrition components of marathon and half-marathon preparation to go off course between day one and race day.

I always breathe a sigh of relief when I start my prerace taper. If I make it that far without getting injured or burning out from overtraining, I know I will make it to the start line fit and healthy because all the hard work has been done. When I get through step four of the taper diet—carbo loading—I feel even more hopeful, because I know I've taken advantage of almost every nutritional opportunity

DESIGNING YOUR TAPER DIET

There are fifty-four different possible taper diets. Only one of these possibilities is the ideal taper diet for your next marathon or half marathon. Despite the wealth of options, finding the ideal taper diet for your next race is not difficult if you approach the selection process methodically. Here's how to do it.

1. Reduce your calorie intake so that you don't gain weight as a result of tapering your training. Reduce your calorie intake three weeks before race day if you're doing a three-week taper, two weeks before race day if you're doing a two-week taper, and one week before race day if you're doing a one week taper.

2. Switch to a 65 percent fat diet two weeks before race day if (a) your initial three-day fat-loading test goes well, (b) you are confident that you can eat a high-fat diet for ten days without unbearable mental anguish, (c) your upcoming race will last more than two hours, and (d) you are tapering for at least two weeks. Alternatively, start a compressed, five-day fat-loading period six days before competition if conditions (a) and (c) are met but you'd rather not fat load for ten days or you're only tapering for one week. Forgo fat loading altogether if your test does not go well, or your upcoming race is shorter than two hours, or you're not comfortable with the idea of getting 65 percent of your calories from fat for even five days.

3. Remove all caffeine from your diet one week before race day if you normally consume caffeine daily in small to moderate amounts and you intend to ingest caffeine on race morning for the sake of performance enhancement. Consider a longer caffeine fast of up to two weeks if you normally consume caffeine daily in large amounts and you think you can bear going without caffeine that long. Skip the caffeine fast altogether if you do not normally consume caffeine or if you do not plan to ingest caffeine before your race.

4. Carbohydrate load. If you choose to fat load for ten days starting two weeks before your race, then switch to a diet that supplies carbs in the amount of 70 percent of total calories for the last three full days before the race. If you fat load for five days beginning one week before your race, then eat 10 g of carbohydrate for every kilogram you weigh on the day before your race. If you don't fat load at all you may choose either the one-day or the three-day carbo load. You can skip carbo loading entirely before races lasting less than two hours.

to enhance my race performance and avoided almost all of the nutritional mistakes that could wreck my performance.

Notice I said "almost." Things can still go off course in the last twenty-four hours before a marathon or half marathon, and often do. Prerace nutrition is the next critical component of performance nutrition.

PRERACE NUTRITION

CHAPTER 6

T he final twelve hours before a marathon or half marathon are the most nutritionally important period in the entire race-preparation process. Much of what you put into your body within this window of time will still be there when the race starts, and thus it will have a significant effect on the outcome of your race. If you put the right things in your body, the effect will be positive, and you will perform much better than you would if you failed to take advantage of the nutritional opportunities that exist in this moment. If you put the wrong things in your body, the effect will be negative—perhaps even disastrous.

The ultimate prerace nutrition nightmare is food poisoning, which is not as rare as you might think. Two days before the 2006 New York City Marathon, for example, Meb Keflezighi ate a bad plate of chicken fettuccine—his standard prerace meal. Unable to eat much in the remaining thirty-six hours before the marathon, Meb struggled to a twentieth-place finish in a race he had hoped to win (and would win three years later with a healthy stomach).

If it seems that these sorts of extreme nutritional catastrophes occur more often before races than before training runs, it's because they do. The reason is that runners are often far from home when they participate in marathons and half marathons and find themselves eating in unfamiliar places and losing some of their customary control over their diet.

Familiarity and *control* are the fundamental principles of effective prerace nutrition. Applying these principles will not only help you avoid food poisoning but will also enable you to avoid the more common types of prerace nutrition problems and take full advantage of the important fueling opportunities that are available before competition. Familiarity is about making a well-rehearsed routine of your prerace fueling, a routine that you repeat with minimal variation before every important race. Control is about knowing exactly what you should and should not do nutritionally in the final twelve hours before a race, and knowing what works best for you individually.

DINNER

Your dinner on the day before a marathon or half marathon is likely to be the last full or "normal" meal you consume prior to racing. The early start times of most races make it difficult to eat a large meal on race morning. The primary objective of your race-eve dinner is to complete the job of carbohydrate loading that was started either that morning or two days earlier (depending on whether you're doing a one-day carbo load after a five-day fat load or a three-day carbo-load after a ten-day fat load). In addition to being high in carbohydrate your prerace dinner should also be relatively low in fat, protein, and fiber. In the case of a one-day carbo load, calculate the amount of carbohydrate in this meal to ensure that you reach your goal of 10 g of carbs per kilogram of body weight for the day. In the case of a three-day carbo load, calculate the amount of carbohydrate in this meal to ensure that you meet your goal of getting 70 percent of your total calories for the day from carbs.

If, for whatever reason, you have neglected to carbo load up to this point and you want to gain what advantage you can from this one meal, your best bet is to choose for your prerace dinner foods that are almost pure carbohydrate. Pasta, rice, potatoes, bread, and certain soups (e.g., tomato) are familiar dinner foods that get almost all of their calories from carbs. Don't overeat for the sake of getting in a few extra grams of carbohydrate. You can get a helpful amount of carbs from a normal-size meal comprising these foods (and perhaps washed down with fruit juice); overeating will only increase your chances of sleeping poorly or having bathroom issues the next morning.

On that same score, avoid eating a late dinner if you can. An earlier dinner increases the likelihood that you will be able to void most of the indigestible materials in the meal the following morning (an act that my sophomoric side likes to refer to as "last-minute weight loss"). Whether your race begins very early (as in the case of the San Francisco Marathon and Half Marathon, whose first waves launch at 5:30 AM), or on the late side (as in the case of the Boston Marathon, whose three waves launch between 10:00 and 10:40 AM), you'll want to sit down for supper around 6:00 PM the evening before.

I like to have a glass of wine or beer with my race-eve dinner. Although I usually avoid alcohol throughout race week as a way to prevent taper-period weight gain, I break my prohibition at the last supper because it helps me relax. I'm not alone; lots of runners who normally enjoy a drink with dinner also do so before races. Deena Kastor, for example, drank a glass of red wine the night before she won a bronze medal in the 2004 Olympic Marathon, and repeated the ritual before setting an American record of 2:19:36 at the Chicago Marathon in 2006.

If you sleep in your own bed the night before a race, you can eat at home, prepare your own dinner, and enjoy total control over what you eat. In this case I would suggest that you eat something you've eaten many times before with good results. It could be a special meal that you reserve for races—such as masters marathon champion Heidy Lozano's "lucky sandwich"—or a menu you prepare frequently before long training runs. Eating at home the night before a race offers no guarantee against digestive problems, though. Lozano unwittingly used tainted meat in her lucky sandwich the night before the 2011 Houston Marathon and was unable to defend her masters title from the previous year. Minimize the risk of such setbacks by checking expiration dates, thoroughly washing vegetables, thoroughly cooking meats, and avoiding raw foods of all kinds (including raw vegetables such as salads) as much as possible in your race-eve dinner.

It's harder to minimize risks when you're forced to eat out the night before a race away from home, but there are some things you can do. First, avoid raw foods just as you would at home. Second, base your meal on foods that are less commonly tainted, such as pastas (it wasn't the fettuccine but the chicken that felled Keflezighi) and other grain-based foods, which also happen to provide the carbs you're seeking. And third, try to eat at more upscale restaurants that are likely to have higher standards for food quality and hygiene.

Eating something that just doesn't agree with you is a more likely occurrence than eating something that actually poisons you, when you have your prerace dinner on the road. The best way to minimize this risk is to try to eat the same thing before every race. For example, no matter which city she's in, Deena Kastor always books a reservation at the best Italian restaurant she can find and eats pasta with pesto sauce and fish—and a glass of wine.

Marathon world record holder Paula Radcliffe of Great Britain is even more cautious. Although she describes herself as an adventurous eater under normal circumstances, the night before a marathon she sups on plain brown rice with chicken.

SLEEP

Once you've packed away your race-eve dinner, your next priority is, of course, sleep. Many runners often find it difficult to get a decent night's sleep before a race because they're nervous, they're probably facing an early wake up, and they may be away from home. Sleeping a little less, or somewhat less soundly, than normal will not ruin your race, especially if you get a full night's sleep the previous night, which you should make happen by any means necessary. But even if you enjoy eight solid hours of shut-eye two nights before your race, a truly sleepless final night will ruin your race. I make sure that poor sleep does not ruin my important races by taking a sleep aid before bed. I recognize that this might not qualify as a nutritional tip, but since sleep aids are things that you put in your body through your mouth, I think it can be counted as one.

If, like many runners, you prefer to minimize the number of drugs you put in your body, you can take a natural sleep aid such as valerian root or melatonin. If you just want to be knocked out in the most effective way possible, get your hands on a prescription sleep medication such as Ambien before your race. You must actually suffer from occasional insomnia between races to get a prescription for such medications, but over-the-counter sleep aids such as Unisom or Tylenol Simply Sleep also work very well for many people. I myself use over-the-counter sleep aids and swear by them. Not only do I sleep better before races when I use them, but I also worry less about getting a good night's rest before I go to bed. Whether you choose a natural sleep aid, a prescription sleep medication, or an over-the-counter product, be sure to test it in training and prior to lower-priority races before you use it on the eve of an important marathon or half marathon.

BREAKFAST

If your race-eve dinner is the last full or normal meal you eat before a race, breakfast on race morning is the last meal of any description that you eat before the starting horn sounds. The sole purpose of this meal is to top off your body's carbohydrate supplies—particularly your liver glycogen stores, which, as I've mentioned before, are typically half-depleted after the overnight fast—without increasing the risk of stomach upset during your event. The ideal meal for this purpose is one that is easy to prepare, eat, and digest, as well as high in carbohydrate and low in protein, fat, and fiber.

Eat your breakfast between four and two hours before the start of your race. If you eat any earlier you may be hungry again and experiencing declining energy levels when it's time to start running. If you eat any later you may still have food in your stomach when it's time to start running. A meal eaten four hours out should be fairly large, providing as much as 4 g of carbohydrate per kilogram of body weight. If you eat two hours before a race your breakfast should be smaller, supplying 1 to 3 g of carbs per kilogram of body weight.

There is a great deal of individual variation in the amount of food that runners are comfortable eating before a race. If you have a high tolerance, take advantage of it by packing in the carbs. Jason Hartmann is one such runner. He ate four bagels and a banana before the start of the 2012 Boston Marathon, where he finished fourth as the top American.

Some runners are unable to eat anything on the morning of an event without suffering gastrointestinal consequences during the race. One might assume that such runners are doomed to hit the wall, at least in full marathons, but this is not the case. Libbie Hickman was never able to eat a prerace breakfast during her stellar competitive running career in the 1990s and that did not stop her from running a 2:28:34 marathon. Among currently active elite runners, Serena Burla is unable to take in anything besides water before longer races and that hasn't stopped her from running an almost identical 2:28:27 marathon.

The key to avoiding the wall in longer races despite not eating beforehand is taking in plenty of carbohydrate during the race. Research has shown that runners experience no major performance decline when they start long time trials in a fasted state, provided they consume carbs at close to the maximum absorption rate of 60 to 90 g per hour during the run. By all means, eat a high-carb breakfast if you can, but if you can't, don't assume you're running with a major disadvantage.

Table 6.1 presents my choices for the five best foods to eat (or drink) before a race. Most of them do not provide all of the carbs you will need in your prerace breakfast, so it may be necessary to eat more than one item, or more than one serving of a single item, or to supplement your chosen food with a high-carb beverage. If you are inclined to pay attention to the glycemic index you will observe that all of these breakfast choices are moderate- to high-glycemic foods— that is, foods whose carbohydrate content is metabolized quickly, causing a rapid rise in blood sugar. High-glycemic foods are widely viewed as "bad" because the energy they supply to the body is not as steady and long-lasting as the energy provided by moderate- and low-glycemic foods. Indeed, some studies have shown that runners perform better after eating a moderate- or low-glycemic meal than they do after eating a high-glycemic meal. But in these studies the various meals have been consumed just forty-five minutes before exercise—close enough that the carbs they contain are still being absorbed. In a more realistic study where a larger meal was consumed three hours before running

TABLE 6.1 *THE 5 BEST PRERACE BREAKFAST FOODS*

FOOD	CARBOHYDRATE CONTENT	ADVANTAGES	DISADVANTAGES
BAGEL	56 g	• Very high in carbs • Familiar breakfast food • Easy to prepare, eat, and digest	• Chewy, which exacerbates prerace nerves in some runners
BANANA	30 g	• High in carbs • Travel friendly • Very easy to eat	• Not as high in carbs as some alternatives
ENERGY BAR (e.g., Power-Bar)	45 g	• Very high in carbs • Zero preparation	• Chewy • Too much protein, fat, and fiber for some runners
MEAL REPLACEMENT DRINK (e.g., Boost)	40 g	• High in carbs • Easy to consume on a nervous stomach	• Not very filling • Too much protein, fat, and fiber for some runners
OATMEAL	30 g	• Very high in carbs • Familiar breakfast food • Easy to eat and digest • Filling	• Requires preparation

to allow time for full absorption of its carbohydrate content, the glycemic index of the meal had no effect on performance. I believe that high-glycemic foods such as those in Table 6.1 are generally *better* choices as prerace breakfast foods simply because higher-glycemic foods typically contain *more* carbohydrate and less protein, fat, and/ or fiber.

Once you find a prerace breakfast that works for you, stick with it. Remember, the two key principles of prerace nutrition are familiarity and control. The comfort you get from eating a ritual breakfast that you're confident in is as important as eating the right kind of breakfast.

Leonard "Buddy" Edelen, a great American marathoner of the early 1960s, learned the hard way not to experiment with his prerace breakfast. On the morning of his very first marathon, a friend of Edelen who was also racing offered him a tin of sardines. It so happened that sardines were a familiar prerunning food for Edelen's friend, and one he had confidence in. Not so for Edelen, but he ate them anyway. The writer Frank Murphy described the consequences in his biography of Edelen, *A Cold Clear Day*: "By six miles Buddy was catching sardines on the way up; in doing so he became nauseous and cramped; nauseous and cramped, his legs went out from underneath him. As his legs went out, he slowed; as he slowed, he grew discouraged; as he grew discouraged, he slowed."

Prior to the 2012 Olympic trials marathons, *Runner's World* asked several of the top contenders what they planned to eat for breakfast on race morning. Among the answers given there were many commonly named items and a few idiosyncratic choices. Deena Kastor (who finished sixth in the race) said she planned to eat eggs on toast and a banana with coffee. Brett Gotcher (fifth) would eat oatmeal, toast, and a banana, as would Desiree Davila (second), minus the banana. Kara Goucher (third) planned to eat toast with coffee. Shalane Flanagan (first) would eat oatmeal, bread, and a banana and drink Gatorade. Ryan Hall (second) would not eat anything but would get plenty of carbs from a shake made with Muscle Milk protein powder and Cytocarb, a powdered drink mix. The most noteworthy shared quality of these various menus was their definiteness. All of these great runners knew exactly what they were going to eat (and exactly when—each runner named a specific breakfast time that fell between three and a half and two hours before the start of the race).

It takes time for many runners to discover the prerace breakfast routine that is ideal for them. If you haven't found yours yet, you may need to experiment. Trying out different breakfasts before Simulator runs and other long workouts can be helpful, but race days are the true tests because prerace nerves affect food preferences and tolerances. Conduct your prerace meal experimentation within the guidelines I've provided, and once you have it dialed in, don't pull a Buddy Edelen by engaging in a spontaneous experiment on marathon morning!

PRERACE HYDRATION

If you've been a runner longer than a week, then you've probably read the following statement at least once, if not dozens of times: "As little as 2 percent dehydration will have a negative effect on your performance." But if this is true, then how can it also be true that, as we saw in Chapter 4, the typical winner of a major marathon is nearly 9 percent dehydrated at the finish line and is still running as fast as he was in the first mile?

The apparent contradiction between these two facts arises from the format of the studies upon which the claim that 2 percent dehydration hurts performance is based. In these studies dehydration is induced through passive heat exposure prior to a bout of exercise. When a person *begins* an exercise test 2 percent dehydrated or more, a negative effect on performance is seen compared to when the same person starts the same test fully hydrated. Things are different, however, when a person begins an exercise test fully hydrated and gradually becomes 2 percent dehydrated or more as a result of drinking less fluid than is lost through perspiration. In these cases, as we have seen, dehydration has no effect on performance as long as the person drinks enough to satisfy his or her thirst.

In short, the often-cited "2 percent dehydration" claim is misleading. But it does make the valuable point that it is important not to be *already dehydrated* when you begin exercise—especially when that exercise is a marathon or half marathon. One of the important objectives of prerace nutrition therefore is ensuring that this doesn't happen.

Few runners start marathons and half marathons in a state of 2 percent dehydration, or even 1 percent. In fact, many runners are overzealous in their prerace hydrations habits. They attempt to "load up" on fluid, drinking much more than they normally do, in the hope that attaining a state of maximal hydration before the race start will minimize the effects of dehydration on their performance in the final miles of the race. This is not a practice that runners have come up with on their own; rather, it is one that they have been taught by coaches and sports nutritionists, some of whom even invoke the famous "pee rule." The running blogger Dave Munger has observed, "One piece of advice I've heard given to marathoners is that you should prehydrate as much as possible before a race: According to this line of reasoning, the more you pee, the better you'll do, and make sure you've had enough that your urine stream is completely clear."

What the runners receiving this advice usually don't know is that it is part of a sports-drink marketing program. Many of the coaches and nutritionists who encourage runners to "prehydrate as much as possible" before races received their own education on preexercise hydration from sources such as the 1996 position statement on exercise and hydration authored by the American College of Sports Medicine. The ACSM is the world's largest and most respected exercise science institution. At the time when this position statement was published, the ACSM was backed by two "Platinum Level" corporate sponsors: Gatorade and the Gatorade Sports Science Institute.

The mere fact that the advice to load up on fluid before races comes through an interested party does not guarantee that it is bad advice—but, in fact, it is bad advice. We have seen that the only thing you're likely to accomplish by drinking as much as possible during races is to increase your risk for GI distress. Similarly, the only thing you'll accomplish by drinking excessively before a race is to increase the number of bathroom trips you need to make before and during the race. Humans are not camels. Our body has minimal capacity to store extra fluid. Any fluid you take in beyond the amount that is required to attain euhydration (normal hydration) will go straight to your bladder. Unless you have allowed yourself to become severely dehydrated over the course of the day and night before your race, you will not need much fluid to attain euhydration on race morning. Twelve to 16 ounces consumed between the time you wake up and one hour before the start of your race should do the trick. If you urinate at least once after your initial visit to the bathroom upon waking up, consider your mission accomplished.

Tim Noakes, author of *Waterlogged: The Serious Problem of Overhydration in Endurance Sports*, advises athletes to stop drinking two hours before the start of a race. I prefer to wait until one hour prior to the gun to stop drinking. I find the two-hour cutoff to be impractical, as I'm often just waking up two hours before race time, and as long as I don't drink too much before, the one-hour cutoff suffices to eliminate the need for midrace bathroom breaks. Many runners who don't realize that they are not camels continue to drink until minutes before the race begins, a behavior that makes about as much sense as drinking a liter of water just before setting out on a long drive toward a destination you're in a hurry to reach.

You can use just about anything you want to hydrate on race morning: water, juice, a sports drink, or some sort of liquid meal. The only bad choices are alcoholic beverages, for obvious reasons, and caffeinated drinks, because they're diuretic and because pure caffeine pills are the best source of prerace caffeine. (I'll talk more about caffeine and caffeine pills in a bit.)

BEET JUICE, ANYONE?

Within the past couple of years I've switched from water to beet juice for prerace hydration. I know it sounds weird, but it has a benefit that is lacking in any other hydration choice and I encourage all runners to try it. Beet juice is rich in dietary nitrates, which are precursors for nitric oxide, a chemical that the body uses to cause blood vessels to dilate. Consuming beet juice before exercise increases vasodilatation and blood flow and reduces the oxygen cost of exercise. These effects translate directly into better race performance, even in highly trained endurance athletes. A 2011 study conducted by researchers at the University of Exeter found that consuming half a liter of beet juice 2.5 hours before cycling time trials of 4 km and 16.1 km improved performance by 2.8 percent and 2.7 percent, respectively, in club-level cyclists.

Beet juice is typically sold in half-liter bottles, which is the perfect amount for prerace hydration. Drink the whole bottle with your prerace breakfast between three and two hours before the gun. Of course, be sure to try it in training before using it on the day of an important race. It doesn't taste great to some people, but who cares how it tastes if it gives you a 2.8 percent performance lift? The only side effect is beet-colored urine for the next several hours. I've also found that beet juice causes mild akathisia, or inner restlessness, which is not a bad thing before a race. Look for beet juice at your local natural foods market.

HOT DAY? TRY A SLUSHIE

Most marathons and half marathons do not take place in hot weather, but if you ever do run a long race on a hot day, there is a special alternative to the usual methods of hydration that you might try. Research has shown that hydrating with a blended ice drink, or slushie, enhances performance during prolonged running in the heat by lowering core body temperature and perceived heat stress. In 2011, Rodney Siegel and colleagues at Australia's Edith Cowan University fed either a syrup-flavored slushie (30°F) or cold water (39°F) to ten male recreational athletes just before they ran to exhaustion on a treadmill in a hot environment (93°F). The athletes were able to run for roughly fifty minutes on average after drinking the slushie, compared to just forty minutes after drinking cold water. Interestingly, slushie ingestion not only delayed the point at which the subjects reached a critically high core body temperature, but also allowed a higher tolerable core body temperature before exhaustion was reached. In other words, the slushie let them start colder *and* get hotter.

If the race-day forecast calls for temperatures above 75°F, find some way to purchase a slushie or blend your own, keep it cold until close to race time, and then drink it. This exception to the one-hour hydration cutoff will do you more good than harm on a hot day by lowering your core body temperature just before you start running.

The most important characteristic of a prerace slushie is temperature—it should be literally ice cold. The slushies used in some studies have been noncaloric—they were sweetened artificially—so clearly this type of formulation is effective, but you can gain additional benefit from a slushie that contains some sugar, as most slushies do. These calories will count toward the final "topping off" of your body's carbohydrate fuel stores.

THE FINAL HOUR

Whether you are participating in a marathon or a half marathon, there is more to be done in the final hour before the start than warming up, being nervous, and making your way to the start area. There are a few nutrition-related priorities left to address within this crucial window. A couple of them, however, are optional.

EMPTYING OUT

As I mentioned earlier, I recommend that you cut off all fluid intake one hour before your scheduled race start time. This will give your

TABLE 6.2 *RACE MORNING NUTRITION TIMELINE*

3 to 2 hours before start	Eat breakfast: 1 to 4 g carbohydrate per kg body weight.
3 hours to 1 hour before start	Hydrate: drink 12 to 16 ounces of water, sports drink, juice, or liquid meal, or (my recommendation) 0.5 L (16.9 ounces) of beet juice.
1 hour before start	Stop drinking: take 3 to 6 mg caffeine per kg of body weight (optional).
30 minutes before start	Take 500 mg of acetaminophen (optional).
2 minutes to 1 minute before start	Consume one 1.2-ounce packet of energy gel or a few gulps (about 4 ounces) of sports drink.

body time to absorb the fluid you've consumed since waking and shunt the excess to your bladder so that you can empty it perhaps twenty or thirty minutes before the gun and start the race with an empty bladder and no worries about needing a bathroom break during the race.

I cannot overstate the importance of doing whatever it takes to minimize the likelihood that you will have to make one or more pit stops during a marathon or half marathon. My friend Kevin Beck learned this lesson the hard way at the 2001 Boston Marathon. He came to the start line in the best shape of his life. Within the first few miles he realized he was having one of those rare, magical days when running fast seems almost effortless. Unfortunately, just a few miles farther down the road he discovered that he needed to use the bathroom. Not "little bathroom," either, as toddlers are taught to say. Big bathroom.

If he'd been having a bad race, Kevin probably would have heeded nature's call right away. But he was on pace for a huge PR, so he pressed on, trying his best to tune out the increasingly urgent complaints of his bowels. Alas, when he reached Cleveland Circle, at 22.5 miles, Kevin no longer had a choice in the matter. He dashed inside a conveniently situated portable toilet and relieved himself. When he dashed back out the huge crowd of spectators that was gathered around the circle erupted in applause and cheering. In the delirium of his fatigue, Kevin thought the people of Boston were congratulating him on his remarkably deft pit stop. Then he realized that the leader of the women's race, Kenya's Catherine Ndereba, had just come through, having been behind him until that point.

Free of his burden, Kevin resumed running and finished only thirty seconds behind Ndereba, setting a new marathon PR of 2:24:25. He wasn't about to grumble, but he also knew that with better timing of his prerace dinner, or better choices of foods for this meal, he might have been forever able to boast of having beaten the first woman in the 2001 Boston Marathon.

The way to avoid such setbacks is to put some thought and planning into taking care of your bathroom needs on race morning. If you don't, you're likely to find yourself stuck in a long Porta Potty line at the last minute and forced to choose between starting late and starting with useless ballast on board your vessel. A variety of tricks can be used to avoid this scenario. One is to get a hotel room within easy walking distance of the start line so you have your own private bathroom at the ready. Another is to choose a warm-up route that takes you to the first set of bathrooms on the actual race course, which usually have short lines or none at all. Some race venues have out-of-the-way or unofficial bathrooms that only veterans of that particular event seem to know about. It can be worthwhile to quiz one or more veterans of your next event on this topic before race day.

CAFFEINE (OPTIONAL)

The last sip of fluid you swallow at the one-hour cutoff should be used to wash down your prerace caffeine pills, if you choose to use them. Caffeine levels in the bloodstream peak one hour after caffeine consumption, so if you take your NoDoz or Stay Awake tablets one hour before your race begins you will be feeling the full effects just as you start to run. Caffeine pills are preferable to coffee for several reasons. First of all, it is simply not practical to have coffee available one hour before the start of a marathon or half marathon, when you're likely to be already at the race site. Even if it were practical to have coffee available at the start line, drinking enough coffee to get the maximum performance benefit just one hour before you started running would almost certainly cause you to require a bathroom break in the middle of the race. Furthermore, research suggests that, for whatever reason, pure caffeine is more effective than coffee as a performance booster. Finally, it's much easier to control your caffeine dosage with pills than it is with coffee.

The optimal dosage of caffeine before exercise has been much researched. A minimum dose of 2 mg of caffeine per kilogram of body weight is required for an ergogenic effect. Doses above 6 mg per kilogram of body weight carry no additional benefit. A 2012 study out of Australia's Griffith University found that a caffeine dose of 3 mg per kilogram of body weight enhanced cycling performance as much as twice that amount. Based on the principle that it's wise not to use more of any drug than is needed to serve its purpose, I suggest that you aim to consume approximately 3 mg of caffeine per kilogram you weigh before your races unless you are normally a heavy caffeine user, in which case a dosage closer to the maximum effective dosage of 6 mg per kilogram may be more effective. Caffeine pills generally come in 200 mg tablets, so you may need to divide tablets to get the right amount. But it's okay to be approximate. A 150-pound (68.2 kg) runner would need to consume 205 mg of caffeine to hit the mark of 3 mg per kilogram. In that case, a single 200 mg would be close enough. Note that if you plan to consume caffeinated energy gels during the race (a topic I'll revisit in the next chapter), you should take somewhat less than the maximum effective dosage before the race so that the total amount of caffeine you take before and during the race does not exceed 6 mg per kilogram of body weight.

ACETAMINOPHEN (OPTIONAL)

Thirty minutes before your race you may wish to take one more pill: namely, a 500 mg dose of acetaminophen, an analgesic (pain-blocking) drug that is best known as the active ingredient in Tylenol. While runners commonly use over-the-counter pain medications to deal with muscle soreness after a marathon or half marathon, research has demonstrated that pre-exercise ingestion of acetaminophen enhances performance by reducing pain during exercise. While every runner knows that racing is painful, most runners do not think of race pain as a performance limiter. But it is. Studies have shown that drugs such as naloxone (which is used to treat overdoses of heroin and morphine and actually increases the perception of pain during exercise) reduce performance even though they do not affect an athlete's physical capacity. On the flip side, performance is enhanced by drugs or other influences that affect perception of effort without affecting any other part of the body besides the brain. In fact, this is precisely how caffeine boosts performance. It does not act on the muscles; it acts on the brain, making running feel easier so that the runner can sustain a faster pace at his or her limit of pain tolerance.

Acetaminophen works in the same way. In a 2008 study, researchers at the University of Bedfordshire, England, gave acetaminophen to ten cyclists before they completed a simulated 10-mile time trial. On average, they completed this time trial 30 seconds (or 2 percent) faster after taking the drug than when they performed the same test after taking a placebo. The cyclists' ratings of perceived exertion were the same in both trials. This finding suggests that the drug reduced the degree of effort that the subjects perceived at their normal time-trial intensity, allowing them to pedal harder at the maximal tolerable level of perceived effort.

Despite these results, some experts discourage the use of acetaminophen before races on the grounds that it could mask the pain of an injury, thereby causing the athlete to continue and exacerbate the problem when he or she ought to stop. I find this scenario implausible. Acetaminophen just isn't that powerful. In the context of a half marathon or marathon it really works by making the overall effort of running feel a bit easier, not by numbing damaged tissues. I have used Tylenol before several marathons and have felt just as sore and beat-up at the end of these races as I have at the end of other marathons. But if the results of the Bedfordshire study are valid, I have completed the Tylenol-assisted races 2 percent faster than I would have done otherwise.

The use of acetaminophen before races is also objected to in some quarters on the grounds that it is being used as a performance-enhancing drug in these circumstances, albeit a legal and (almost certainly safe) one. But again, caffeine, whose use before and during competition almost no one objects to, is also a drug and works in a very similar way. While I have no ethical or safety concerns about taking Tylenol before races, I respect those who do, so I do not actively advise runners to follow my example in this regard. I merely present it as an option. If it's an option you wish to try, test it in training before you use it in a race situation.

TOPPING OFF

The very last step in prerace nutrition is reserved for one or two minutes before the gun, when you're already on the start line. At this time I suggest that you swallow a packet of energy gel (with or without a bit of water) or a few gulps of sports drink. Because this nutrition is just beginning to be absorbed into the body when you get going, it really counts as the first step in race fueling. And as race fueling is the topic of the next chapter, I'll further explain this nutritional measure there.

RACE NUTRITION

The human body is not designed to absorb food or drink while running. That's because eating and drinking on the run are very new behaviors for our species—something we started doing in earnest a few decades ago and *never* did for about two million years prior to that time. Anthropologists believe that early humans did lots of long-distance running, but our ancient ancestors had no way of drinking as they ran—no squeeze bottles or CamelBaks to suck from—and because most of the running they did was in fight-or-flight situations, eating had to wait until after the task was completed. There was no survival advantage associated with being able to drink or eat while running, for the simple reason that nobody ever did it. Thus, although early humans underwent many evolutionary adaptations that made them better runners, they did not evolve in ways that made them better able to eat or drink on the run.

This evolutionary inheritance can be clearly observed today in the physiological effects of running on our digestive system. When we start to run our body shunts blood flow away from the digestive organs to the muscles, impeding the breakdown and absorption of food. Hormonal changes cause appetite to disappear and slow the digestion of anything that is consumed. The faster we run, the slower the stomach empties. And to cap it all off, the sloshing of the stomach contents that occurs during running causes feelings of discomfort similar to those experienced by a kid who rides a roller coaster after eating a Coney Island hot dog.

Together these factors add up to a simple message from our body to our conscious faculties: *Do not eat or drink while running.* We can disregard this message to some degree without suffering ill effects. But drinking or eating more than a modest amount while running is almost certain to cause debilitating gastrointestinal symptoms.

On the other hand, drinking (and perhaps also eating) a tolerable amount of the right stuff enhances performance in marathons and half marathons. To eat and drink nothing therefore is to needlessly limit one's performance. Optimal race nutrition is a balancing act. The object is to consume enough of the right stuff to push back the wall of fatigue but not so much of anything that bloating, sloshing, nausea, or worse causes you to slow down.

One trick that helps with this balancing act is beginning the race-fueling process before the race itself starts, as I suggested at the conclusion of the previous chapter. To get a meaningful performance benefit from carbohydrate during a race you need to consume at least 30 g of carbohydrate per hour. Drinking roughly 4 ounces of a sports drink or swallowing one packet of energy gel a few minutes before the race starts will contribute 10 to 25 g of carbs toward this quota. Because these carbs will not enter your bloodstream until you're already running, they count as race nutrition. But because this nutrition is ingested while you're still at rest, it will be less likely to contribute toward later GI problems than will an equal amount of sports drink or gel consumed within the race.

This little "cheat" is something that almost every runner—even those with a sensitive stomach—can and should exploit at the beginning of every marathon and half marathon. From this point, however, the race plans of individual runners must necessarily diverge. There is no single race nutrition plan that works best for every runner in every race. Different plans work best for different bodies. There are five general marathon and half-marathon fueling strategies to choose from. The strategy that fits you best depends primarily on your tolerance for fluid and energy intake while racing.

5 MARATHON AND HALF-MARATHON FUELING STRATEGIES

If you ask a dozen experienced runners to describe their marathon and half-marathon nutrition plans, you're likely to get a dozen different answers. But some of the differences are sure to be small details, such as preferred flavors of energy gels. If you compare individual race nutrition plans at the most substantive level, you will find that there are only five general strategies that experienced runners commonly employ.

All of these strategies are used in both marathons and half marathons, but not always by the same runner. Many runners find that the fueling plan that works best for them in marathons is different from the plan that works best in half marathons. Generally, runners are not able to consume fluid and energy at as high a rate in half marathons because of the higher intensity. Fortunately, most runners also do not *need* to take in as much fluid and carbohydrate in half marathons because less total fluid is lost and less muscle glycogen is burned.

With few exceptions, elite runners who are able to complete half marathons in less than 75 minutes consume nothing. Research has shown that hydration and carbohydrate intake provide no performance benefit to the fittest athletes in races that last less than this amount of time, and any small advantage an elite runner might get from drinking during a half marathon is usually negated by the difficulty and disruptiveness of trying to drink while running 10.5 mph or faster.

If you're a runner who takes between eighty minutes and two hours to complete a half marathon you may or may not be able to tolerate the same rate of fluid and energy intake in half marathons as you do in marathons. In any case, you can expect to maximize your performance by drinking according to your thirst (and stomach comfort) and getting at least 30 g of carbohydrate per hour. If you require more than two hours to complete a half marathon, you should be able to practice the same nutrition plan in these races that you use in marathons. Note, however, that in many half marathons aid stations are more spread out than they are in marathons, so you may have to tweak your plan regardless.

The following five race nutrition plans are ranked in order of preferability for races lasting longer than two hours. Race Nutrition Plan #1 is the easiest way to get the optimal amounts of fluid and carbohydrate for maximum performance, so you should use it if you can. Not every runner can, in which case Race Nutrition Plan #2 is the next best alternative, and so on.

PLAN #1: SPORTS DRINK + GELS + WATER

In very long endurance races such as Ironman triathlons and ultramarathons there is an apparent dose-response relationship between carbohydrate intake and performance. In plain English this means that in such races participants who consume more carbs tend to finish faster. It does not mean that every athlete would perform best if he or she consumed as much carbohydrate as the racer who takes in the most carbs in a given race, but at the group level there is a clear correlation between greater carbohydrate intake and better performance.

In shorter races such as 10Ks there is no performance benefit associated with consuming carbs in any amount. Somewhere between sixty and ninety minutes, a threshold is crossed, beyond which taking in some carbohydrate—at least 30 g per hour—is better than taking in none. And somewhere beyond 90 minutes of race duration, a second threshold is crossed, beyond which consuming larger amounts of carbohydrate—at least 60 and up to 90 g per hour—is better than taking in less. Alex Hutchinson, who writes the "Sweat Science" blog for runnersworld.com, speculates that this second threshold probably falls just below the marathon distance for most runners. If he's right, then runners should try to consume close to the maximum amount of carbohydrate they can tolerate during marathons.

The trouble is that, above a certain level, increased carbohydrate intake elevates the risk of GI distress more than it enhances performance. Many runners cannot stomach 60 g of carbs per hour. To determine your personal tolerance you will need to experiment with various rates of carbohydrate intake within race-simulation workouts

WHAT THE PROS DO

Elite runners are good role models for other runners in many respects. The things they tend to do are the things that tend to work; after all, professional runners have a lot more at stake than do the rest of us in their training and racing, and if the tools and methods they used did not work, then they wouldn't be elite runners in the first place. But it is not possible for age-group runners to emulate everything that elite runners do. For example, elite runners are given their own special aid stations in races, where they are allowed to place fluid bottles filled with whatever they choose. Age-group runners, on the other hand, must either drink the official sports drink given out at aid stations for the masses or carry their own fluid.

It is interesting to note that virtually all elite runners fill their bottles with some kind of sports drink. Very few of them drink water. Why would they, when sports drinks provide both of the major performance-enhancing nutrients—water and carbohydrate? An elite runner who chose to hydrate with water in races would have to rely on energy gels entirely to supply carbohydrate. Almost none of them actually do this because sports drinks generally sit a little more comfortably in the stomach than energy gels. Elite runners with stronger stomachs therefore rely on sports drinks to supply most of their carbohydrate (and all of their fluid) and use energy gels to supply the balance of their carbohydrate needs. (In other words, they practice Race Nutrition Plan #1; see page 136.) Elite runners with a more sensitive stomach typically consume sports drinks only in races—eschewing gels and water—because they find that sports drinks supply as much carbohydrate as they can tolerate in the most efficient way. Sure, there are some sports drinks that certain runners cannot tolerate, but there is at least one sports drink that works for most runners, and because elite runners have total freedom to choose their favorite, it makes no sense not to do so, whether they supplement it with gels or not.

While the race nutrition strategies of most elite runners are the same in their general outlines, the details vary from one runner to the next based on the results of each runner's personal experimentation. For example, Stephanie Rothstein, a 2:29 marathoner who trains with the Adidas McMillan Elite team in Flagstaff, Arizona, drinks Gatorade at odd-numbered aid stations and consumes between one-half and two-thirds of a PowerGel with water at even-numbered aid stations. (Elite aid stations are located at 5K intervals in most marathons.) Dathan Ritzenhein drinks 6 ounces of Gatorade with energy gels mixed in at each aid station.

and actual races. If you discover that you can comfortably consume more than 60 g of carbs per hour during prolonged efforts at race intensity, count yourself fortunate and consider limiting yourself to 60 g per hour in marathons nevertheless. The advantage to be gained by taking in more is smaller than the inherent risk, and because of the unique stressfulness of racing, carbohydrate tolerance is typically a little lower in races than in workouts.

Among the most successful marathon runners there are very few who consume more than 60 g of carbohydrate per hour, but there are some. Dathan Ritzenhein, whose marathon nutrition plan I described earlier, takes in as much as 90 g of carbohydrate per hour in marathons, which represents the maximum rate of carbohydrate absorption during running in humans. He was not always able to tolerate such a high rate of energy intake, but trained his stomach to accept it over time. So there is precedent for this level of fuel ingestion in marathons. Hence, if you have a strong stomach and you seem to benefit from levels of carbohydrate intake above 60 g per hour in race-simulation runs, feel free to experiment with the "Ritzenhein Method" in a race.

As I first mentioned in Chapter 4, it is impractical to get 60 g of carbs per hour exclusively from the sports drink offered on the course. Cytomax, for example, is the official sports drink of many marathons and half marathons. To get 60 g of carbohydrate through Cytomax alone you would have to drink almost 33 ounces. The only way most runners could do that would be to slow down so much (for the sake of reducing stomach jostling and increasing the gastric emptying rate) as to defeat the very purpose of maximizing their carbohydrate intake.

Assuming that the sports drink that is available in a given race is one that contains a useful amount of carbohydrate and does not upset your stomach, the best way to get 60 g of carbohydrate per hour is to rely on the sports drink to supply most of your fluid and carbohydrate needs and use energy gels to supply the balance of your carbohydrate needs. To determine how much carbohydrate you're likely to get from the official sports drink, you need to know how many grams of carbs are provided in 1 ounce of the product and how many aid stations on the racecourse will be stocked with it. The Chicago Marathon, to cite a concrete case, is typical of today's major marathons in providing twenty aid stations, or one aid station every 1.3 miles. The sports drink offered at the 2012 Chicago Marathon was Gatorade, which supplies 1.75 g of carbohydrate per ounce. Some smaller events do not post detailed aid station information online. In those cases you'll need to contact the event organizer and ask.

Remember that my advice for hydration during running is to drink according to your thirst. In training, when you're carrying your own fluid, you will do this by drinking literally whenever you feel like it. In a race, however, you can only drink when you pass an aid station. Thus in races you're not drinking by thirst so much as you are drinking by feel, or comfort. Because you are likely to perform better if you drink at close to the highest rate that is comfortable for you, I recommend that you try to drink something at every aid station. If you're not very thirsty or feel that your stomach could only tolerate a small sip at any given aid station, take a sip. If you're thirstier or feel your tummy could tolerate more, drink more.

The average amount of sports drink in the paper or plastic cups handed out at aid stations is 4 ounces. A runner who drinks one such cup at every station—that is, 4 ounces every 1.3 miles—will consume anywhere from 10 to 18 ounces per hour, depending on his or her pace. Research has shown that runners typically consume 13 to 27 ounces per hour when they drink by thirst. This means that most runners can comfortably take in at least one full cup of sports drink per aid station in races. You will need to experiment to determine how much sports drink you are likely to consume per aid station. A good way to start is to measure out 4 ounces and drink it every 1.3 miles in some training runs to see how that treats you. This will also calibrate your sense of how much you're actually drinking at race aid stations.

Let's assume for the sake of illustration that you anticipate drinking 4 ounces of sports drink at each aid station in your next event. Four ounces of Gatorade provide 7 g of carbohydrate. Multiply that by twenty aid stations and you get a total of 140 g of carbs for the race. To determine how many carbs you'll get per hour of running, divide this total by your anticipated finish time. Let's say you're planning to finish the Chicago Marathon in three hours and thirty minutes. This means you'll get (140 ÷ 3.5 =) 40 g of carbs per hour from the sports drink, leaving a balance of 20 g of carbs that you'll need to get from energy gels.

Most marathons provide energy gels only at a single aid station near the 20-mile mark. So if you plan to rely on gels to provide some of the carbs you need to get 60 total g per hour, you'll have to carry your own gels. A typical energy gel contains 25 g of carbs per packet. If you swallowed one packet per hour on top of drinking Gatorade at every aid station you would get 65 g per hour. However, it's best to consume energy gels with water, as washing them down with a sports drink creates a very concentrated carbohydrate load in the stomach that few runners can tolerate. If you drink water instead of Gatorade at one aid station per hour—specifically the aid station at which you consume your hourly gel—you will lose the 3.5 g of carbs you would have gotten from Gatorade. With this substitution you will get 61.5 g of carbs per hour from Gatorade and energy gels combined.

Some runners (myself included) find it difficult to consume a full packet of energy gel at once, even with water. If this is the case for you, empty a few gel packets into a gel flask such as those made by Fluid Belt and wear it in a clip on your shorts. With this tool you can sip smaller amounts of gel more frequently to avoid overloading your stomach. I mix 3.5 ounces of gels with 2.5 ounces of water in a 6-ounce flask to make it more drinkable and even easier on my stomach. I take a small slug from the flask every half hour or so and by doing so I usually empty the flask somewhere between the 20-mile mark and the finish line.

There are many individual variations on this general race nutrition plan. If you apply the basic framework of this plan to a few races you will surely find ways to tweak it so that it works optimally for you. Be sure to test your chosen plan in a Simulator run before each marathon and half marathon as well.

PLAN #2: GELS + WATER

On page 137 I mentioned that nearly all elite runners practice Race Nutrition Plan #1 because they are able to choose any sports drink they like and it's easier to meet combined fluid and carbohydrate needs when a sports drink is used. Nonelite runners are in a different situation. We cannot choose the sports drink that is offered at aid stations. When the sports drink chosen by the race management is unpalatable or is a "low-sugar" pseudo sports drink that lacks adequate carbohydrate, it may be necessary to rely on energy gels exclusively to provide the carbohydrate you need. Race Nutrition Plan #2—energy gels plus water—is the best fit for runners who can tolerate higher amounts of carbohydrate intake in races but who happen to find themselves in races where they cannot exercise the preferable option of Race Nutrition Plan #1—sports drink plus energy gels.

To get 60 g of carbohydrate per hour from a typical energy gel (24 g of carbs per packet), you'll need to swallow one packet every twenty-four minutes or so. Research suggests that between 10 and 20 percent of runners are not able to tolerate this rate of gel intake. If you're among the unlucky minority, then try to get at least 30 g per hour from gels. But before you resort to that, experiment with squeezing gels into a gel flask and perhaps mixing them with a little water (as described on page 140) to see whether consuming smaller amounts of gel more frequently enables you to get 60 g of carbs per hour without serious GI complaints.

And while this next suggestion may just sound like a spin on "suck it up," bear with me. You may just need to learn to put up with some stomach discomfort associated with carbohydrate intake. Many runners assume that any degree of stomach discomfort is unacceptable and harmful to performance. This assumption is incorrect. Studies indicate that runners perform better with higher rates of carb intake in races even when they suffer mild to moderate stomach discomfort. Obviously, there is such a thing as intolerable discomfort, but don't assume that any degree of discomfort is unacceptable. Also remember that, as I mentioned in Chapter 4, other research has shown that higher rates of carbohydrate intake tend to become more comfortable with practice.

As for the water component of the water-plus-gels race nutrition strategy, the principle of drinking according to your thirst applies. Most marathons and half marathons have enough aid stations to supply as much water as any runner would ever drink voluntarily, which is as much as you ever should drink. It is never necessary to carry your own water in a marathon or half marathon.

PLAN #3: SPORTS DRINK ONLY

Relying on a sports drink exclusively for your marathon or half-marathon nutrition will be the best plan for your next race if the official sports drink is acceptable to you and you don't tolerate gels well or can't comfortably take in more carbohydrate than a sports drink alone provides. It is extremely unlikely that you will be able to take in 60 g of carbohydrate per hour with this plan, but if you drink as much as your thirst demands and your stomach's comfort allows then you should get at least 30 g per hour.

Don't fret if you must resort to Race Nutrition Plan #3 instead of either of the first two. You're in good company. Brett Gotcher, a 2:10 marathoner, gets all of his nutrition during races from a sports drink (Xtreme Mango Gatorade, specifically). He tried supplementing this with energy gels in his first marathon, but his stomach rejected them. He now drinks roughly 6 ounces of Gatorade per aid station, which works out to about 34 g of carbs per hour of racing. That's less than the optimal amount of 60 g per hour but above the minimum effective dosage of 30 g per hour.

Because the carbohydrate concentration of sports drinks is much lower than that of energy gels, it is important to drink at the high end of your comfort range if you're relying on a sports drink exclusively in races. It is not uncommon for runners to be able to drink as much as 27 ounces per hour without discomfort if they are highly responsive to their thirst. At that rate (with a standard sports drink) a runner will take in more than 47 g of carbs per hour, which isn't half bad. Be aware that you may have to take more than one 4-ounce cup of sports drink at some aid stations to fully exploit your tolerance for fluid intake (especially if the pouring sizes are smaller). Also note that if you do not consume gels during a race, you should not drink any water either because you don't want to waste an opportunity to take in carbs by quenching your thirst with a fluid that contains none.

Race Nutrition Plan #3 is only viable if the official sports drink of your next race is one that sits well in your tummy and contains at least 10 g of carbs per 8 ounces. If the official sports drink of a race you're considering running is not acceptable and you are unable to tolerate energy gels as an alternative carbohydrate source I suggest you find another event to run. Some runners carry their own sports drink as a workaround in such situations, but it doesn't make much sense. The extra weight slows them down more than the product itself speeds them up. If there's a particular event that you're determined to run even though you don't like the sports drink, that's fine—just don't expect to have your best possible race if you carry your own sports drink or if you drink only water from aid stations and thus take in no carbs at all. Your goal in such races should be to *have* a good time, not to *run* a good time.

If the official sports drink in a given race has an adequate carbohydrate content and sits well in your stomach but you just don't like the flavor, drink it anyway. It's a race, for crying out loud, not a cocktail party! You can drink something that tastes good after you finish.

PLAN #4: WATER ONLY (PLUS SPORTS DRINK MOUTH RINSING)

In 2005 researchers at Maastricht University in the Netherlands compared the effects of water and a sports drink in runners. Ninety-eight runners were asked to complete an 18 km time trial on three separate occasions, drinking water on one occasion and a couple of different sports drink formulations in the other two trials. Severe gastrointestinal complaints were relatively uncommon, but they occurred more frequently with both sports drinks than they did with water. These findings confirm anecdotal reports that some runners are unable to tolerate any amount of carbohydrate intake during running and must therefore completely forgo the benefits of consuming carbs during races.

Or must they? In a series of clever studies, Asker Jeukendrup and colleagues at the University of Birmingham, England, found that runners and cyclists were able to complete time trials faster when they periodically rinsed their mouths with a sports drink and spit it out. Although the sports drink was never swallowed and the carbs in it never reached the athletes' muscles, where they could actually be used to supply energy, those carbs stimulated carbohydrate receptors on the tongue of the athletes, and these receptors in turn delivered signals to a part of the brain that is involved in regulating perceived effort during exercise. Activation of this "reward center" in the brain caused running and cycling to feel easier, enabling the athletes to sustain a faster pace in time trials without exceeding their maximum pain tolerance.

This discovery raises the possibility that runners with sensitive stomachs can enjoy at least some of the benefit of using a sports drink without actually drinking it. If you are unable to ingest any carbohydrate during races without risking severe GI distress, then your optimal race nutrition plan entails drinking water by thirst and rinsing out your mouth with a sports drink. I know it sounds weird, but if you're not using any other source of carbs, tasting and spitting out the event's official sports drink will very likely enable you to finish faster than if you drink only water.

Most aid stations in marathons and half marathons are divided into two sections. Water is offered in the first section and sports drink in the second. If you have made a commitment to execute Race Nutrition Plan #4 in a race, take a cup of water from the first section of each aid station and drink as little or as much of it as your thirst requires and your stomach comfort permits. Then take a cup of sports drink from the second section and rinse your mouth with it, spitting it out instead of swallowing. By merely tasting carbs frequently throughout the race you may get almost as much benefit as you would get from ingesting carbs without putting your stomach under duress.

PLAN #5: NOTHING

The gastrointestinal problems that runners experience during running are generally blamed on the carbohydrates or, less often, the fluids they consume. However, some runners are prone to suffer GI symptoms during strenuous efforts even when they consume nothing at all. While any runner who takes in too much nutrition is likely to encounter a problem, it is evident that an unlucky fraction of runners is innately susceptible to experiencing GI troubles when running. A 2012 study involving 221 endurance athletes found that the strongest predictor of abdominal discomfort during races was prior episodes of the same.

Although runners who have this innate susceptibility may encounter problems regardless of whether they consume nutrition during races, their only chance of minimizing the risk of debilitating problems may be to consume nothing.

Before you give up on drinking during races, experiment a little. If your symptoms are no better when you drink nothing than they are when you do drink a little, you might as well go ahead and drink a little unless your symptoms include stomach sloshing—an indication that your body is not absorbing what you drink. If not drinking is really your only option, then embrace Race Nutrition Plan #5 and take comfort in knowing that 2:07 marathons have been run without the aid of any fluid intake. This is not to say that *you* will run a 2:07 without drinking, but you may be able to achieve your goals despite this small handicap. The key is in training without nutrition intake, which will inure your body to fairly high levels of dehydration and fat reliance so that fluid and fuel deprivation during races does not greet your body as a cruel and unusual stressor.

The percentage of runners who cannot drink at all during marathons and half marathons is small. Most runners, however, encounter moments in races when they cannot take in nutrition comfortably. All runners must listen to their body and be willing to stray from their nutrition plan when the GI system sends warning signals. In the 2011 New York City Marathon Shalane Flanagan swallowed 4 ounces of Gatorade, as planned, at the first aid station. By the time she reached the next aid station those 4 ounces of fluid were still sloshing around in her stomach and causing no small amount of discomfort. Flanagan made a spontaneous decision to skip her second drinking opportunity, and because the problem in her gut never abated, she never drank again through the remainder of the race. Even so, she finished second, becoming the first American woman in twenty years to take the runner-up spot at the New York City Marathon. Had Flanagan lacked the confidence to depart from her nutrition plan she might not have finished at all.

Your race nutrition plan should represent a best-case scenario— what you would like to consume provided your body allows it. Be prepared to take in less at any point if necessary. In marathons, especially, tolerance tends to decline toward the end of the race. Few runners feel like drinking much after 20 miles. If you're able to stick close to your plan through the first 20 miles, consider anything you're able to swallow after that point gravy (so to speak).

PROTEIN POWER

In an earlier chapter I mentioned that, while carbohydrate is the most important energy source in the sports drinks and energy gels that are used during running, protein has its place, too. There is evidence that a little protein taken with carbs during prolonged exercise enhances endurance more than carbohydrate alone. I consume a small amount of protein in my marathons—about 1 g for every 4 g of carbohydrate—and you should consider doing the same.

Most sports drinks and energy gels do not contain protein, but a few do. The original and most popular brand of sports drink with protein, Accelerade, is not offered on the course at many marathons or half marathons. However, Accelerade's maker also sells two brands of energy gel, Accel Gel and 2nd Surge, which you may choose to carry during events. I myself carry 2nd Surge during marathons, choosing it over other gels—and not only because I helped formulate it!

The research comparing the benefits of conventional sports drinks and energy gels that do not contain protein and alternative products that do has been controversial. No study has ever shown that a conventional sports drink or energy gel improved endurance performance more than a protein-powered alternative did. Several studies have shown that a sports drink or energy gel containing protein elevated performance more than a conventional product did. And a few studies have shown no difference.

The rate of carbohydrate intake seems to have a big effect on the results of such studies. When carbs are consumed at a rate of 60 g per hour or greater, the addition of protein seems to have little or no effect on performance. At lower rates of carbohydrate intake, however, the addition of protein provides a big performance boost, even when the total number of calories is held equal between the two products. For reasons that are not yet understood, the addition of a small amount of protein to a sports drink or energy gel seems to increase the effectiveness of its carbohydrate content while also reducing perceived effort. One study even found that a low-calorie protein-enhanced sports drink enhanced endurance performance as much as a conventional sports drink despite containing 55 percent less carbohydrate.

These findings are especially relevant to us runners, who are generally unable to consume as much carbohydrate during competition as athletes in other sports. The use of protein-enhanced energy gels in marathons and half marathons may enable runners to get the level of performance increase associated with consuming 60 g of carbs or more per hour despite actually consuming less. The research suggests that 30 g of carbohydrate consumed per hour of exercise is the functional equivalent of 60 g provided it is accompanied by 7 or 8 g of protein.

If the performance-boosting effect of adding protein to a sports drink or energy gel is slightly cloudy to scientists, another benefit is crystal clear. Research has consistently shown that protein-enhanced sports drinks and energy gels drastically reduce the amount of muscle damage incurred during exercise. I believe that muscle damage is an underestimated contributor to fatigue in marathons and half marathons. Sports drinks and energy gels with added protein may push back the wall another step by protecting the muscles of the lower extremities against the effect of the beating they endure in long races.

Some energy gel makers, including GU and Hammer Gel, are now adding amino acids to their products. Because amino acids are the building blocks of proteins, it is likely that these products offer some of the same advantages as gels with complete proteins in them. However, to my knowledge this has not been demonstrated scientifically.

CAFFEINE DURING THE RACE

We've already gone over the benefits of taking caffeine before the start of a marathon or half marathon. But what about taking caffeine during the race? A number of energy gels contain caffeine. Should you use them?

If the choice is between taking caffeine before a race or during it, you're definitely better off taking it before the race. One reason is that, as I've already mentioned, it takes an hour for caffeine to exert its full effect on the brain after it is consumed. It is also easier and less chancy to take a large dose of caffeine at rest than during strenuous running.

Studies have found that caffeine enhances carbohydrate uptake by the muscles when the two substances are consumed together during exercise. Other research has shown that energy gels that contain caffeine are tolerated about as well as those that do not. So there's no reason *not* to consume caffeinated gels during your half marathons and marathons if you're consuming gels anyway, unless you prefer to avoid caffeine altogether. The energy gel I assisted in formulating, 2nd Surge, contains 100 mg of caffeine per pack in addition to 18 g of carbohydrate and 3 g of protein.

Some runners "save" the use of caffeinated gels for the last few miles of the race, as though supporting a strong finish were all that caffeine was good for. In fact, caffeine can help you run stronger the whole way through your events, so if you're going to use caffeine at all, you might as well use it early and late and in between.

Just don't overuse it. If you do choose to consume caffeine both before and during races, do a little math to ensure that you don't consume more than 6 mg of caffeine per kilogram of body weight in total.

MUSCLE CRAMPS

Joe Lemel's first marathon was the 2008 Chicago Marathon. A fifty-five-year-old homebuilder, Joe had started running eighteen months earlier and trained with a balanced program in which he ran four times a week, used an elliptical trainer twice a week, and lifted weights three times. During the race he drank water and swallowed a packet of GU energy gel every forty minutes. He felt great at the halfway point, which he reached in 2:04:50. But a few miles down the road Joe's calf muscles cramped horribly and he limped to the finish line in 4:45:57, where he joined me and many others in the Wall-Hitters Club.

After the race Joe e-mailed me and asked for advice on how to avoid cramping in his next marathon. He told me he was considering doubling up on his GU intake in his next marathon to prevent the electrolyte depletion that others had suggested was the cause of his cramps and asked whether I thought it was a good idea. I told him it was not.

Muscle cramping is one of the most frustrating causes of hitting the wall in half marathons and, especially, marathons. Many runners believe that muscle cramping is caused by dehydration and/or sodium depletion and thus attempt to prevent it by drinking more and/or by consuming extra sodium, perhaps in the form of salt tablets. But muscle cramping during running is not, in fact, caused by dehydration or sodium depletion and cannot be prevented by means of extra fluid or sodium intake.

Numerous studies have proved that there is no link between the "usual suspects" and muscle cramping. In one such study researchers at North Dakota State University used electrical stimulation to induce cramps in the calf muscles (the most common site of cramping) of subjects before and after they cycled indoors in a hot environment until they were 3 percent dehydrated. The objective was simple: to see whether the calf muscles were more susceptible to cramping when the subjects were dehydrated. Turns out they were not. There was, in fact, no difference in the amount of electrical stimulation required to induce cramping before and after the dehydrating exercise.

So what *does* cause muscle cramping? A growing number of experts now believe that exercise-induced muscle cramps are brought on by a special kind of fatigue. This theory is supported by the fact that cramps always occur in working muscles instead of passive muscles and by the fact that muscle cramping almost always occurs in races, seldom in training. Coupled with certain physiological evidence, these observations suggest that cramping is an abnormal neurological response to extreme muscle fatigue.

The number one predictor of muscle cramping in individual athletes is prior cramping episodes. It seems that some unlucky athletes are especially susceptible to exercise-induced muscle cramps. When a given muscle in such a person is subjected to an unaccustomed extremity of exertion, the nerves controlling that muscle may essentially freak out, causing spasm.

There is no nutritional measure that could possibly prevent such an event from occurring. The best advice I can offer cramp-prone runners is to make the "unaccustomed exertion" of running half marathons and marathons somewhat less unaccustomed by patiently accumulating race experience and by preceding each race with one or two very hard workouts that simulate the exertion of the race as closely as they reasonably can. The idea is to gradually push back the threshold of the onset of cramping, from eight miles to 11 miles to 14 miles and so on, until eventually you can reach the finish line of any race before cramping begins.

Despite the lack of evidence to support the electrolyte-depletion theory of muscle cramping, there are many anecdotal cases of runners who seem to experience a prophylactic effect from consuming salt tablets during long races. I've encountered more than a few athletes who say they don't care what the studies I cite say—they swear that salt tablets prevent cramps. At worst, salt tablets are harmless when used according to product label directions, so if you're a frequent cramper and you're desperate, it can't hurt to try them.

A WORD ON PACING

Nutrition intake during races is not the only factor that can push you beyond the wall. Pacing is equally important. Obviously, the faster you run, the faster your muscle glycogen stores diminish and the sooner you hit the wall. Performance in marathons and half marathons is not always limited by glycogen availability, but more often than not, a runner's optimal race pace is the fastest speed he or she can sustain from the start line to the finish line without running out of glycogen.

It's not enough, however, to *average* your optimal pace. You must also run at a steady pace. The reason is that speeding up from your optimal pace increases glycogen usage more than slowing down decreases it. Therefore you will hit the wall sooner in a race if your pace fluctuates above and below the optimum than you will if your pace is consistent, even if your average pace is the same.

Your goal in every half marathon and marathon should be to maintain as constant a pace as possible. Given factors such as hills and winds, it is not always possible to hold a perfectly steady pace. But you can maintain a consistent *effort* despite such factors, and by doing that you will reach the finish line faster than you will if you race like a yo-yo.

CHAPTER 8

AFTER THE RACE

The hardest marathon I've ever run was the one that came at the end of Ironman Wisconsin in 2002. I'll never forget the panic that seized me as I took the painful first steps of that marathon after having just raced my bike 112 miles and swum 2.4 miles before that. The feeling in my legs was familiar. I had last experienced it at the *finish* of my last marathon. I did not see how I could possibly finish this one.

Somehow I managed to survive the full 26.2 miles. After crossing the finish line and passing through the finishing chute I came upon a table laid out with dozens of fresh, piping-hot pizzas. Without a moment's hesitation I grabbed a slice and gobbled it, as though these pies were the whole point of the previous ten hours and thirteen minutes of suffering. It was obvious to me that whoever had thought to put the pizzas there had done at least one Ironman himself. They were exactly what I needed at that moment.

Some sports nutritionists would beg to differ. The conventional advice for postrace nutrition is to avoid eating fatty foods, such as cheese, because they will slow the absorption of the carbs that are needed to refuel the muscles and the protein that is needed to rebuild

151

them. Runners are also warned against drinking alcohol after races because it interferes with rehydration.

All of this is true. But in my view a runner's body is so ravaged after a long race that it scarcely matters what he or she eats or drinks in the first hours of recovery. Only time and rest—and lots of them—can reverse the damage that's been done. Research has shown that the leg muscles remain significantly weaker than normal five days after a marathon. Muscle damage biomarkers are still elevated more than one week after a marathon. Immune system disturbances persist even longer. The timetable for your physiological recovery after a race will be marginally affected at most by your food and beverage choices at this time. Whether you eat pizza or a salad, or drink beer or a fruit smoothie, you won't be ready for hard running for at least a couple of weeks. The one thing you must do in the first two weeks after a marathon or half marathon is take it easy. What you eat and drink in the first twenty-four hours really doesn't matter very much.

One could even argue that pizza and beer are better choices than salads and smoothies after a hard race. We runners are human beings, after all, not robots. Like everyone else, we enjoy the taste of some foods that are not especially healthy. It takes a lot of discipline to resist most of these foods while preparing for a big race. Indulging in a little bit of unhealthy eating after a race is a natural way to reward that discipline. The prospect of such indulgence also has a way of fortifying your restraint during the training process. Few of us could bear the thought of having to eat more or less perfectly for the rest of our lives without reprieve. Knowing that you will allow yourself to enjoy some pizza and beer (or whatever it is you crave) after completing a race might make it easier for you to maintain high dietary standards through three or four months of focused training.

I think that too many sports nutritionists forget that food affects both our physical health and our psychological health. Sometimes eating in a way that is not in the best interest of our physical health is the best thing for our psychological health. The term *comfort food* captures this idea. The first hours, days, and perhaps even weeks after a big race are a time when it's probably more important to eat for psychological health than for physical health. Unless you're a member of the Marathon Maniacs club who runs a marathon almost every weekend and therefore must do everything possible to recover quickly after each event, you should forget about recovery and eat whatever you want for up to two weeks following the completion of a training cycle. This short period of indulgence will leave you ready to return to disciplined eating in preparation for the next big event in much the same way that a couple of weeks of rest will restore your hunger to train.

RECOVERY NUTRITION

Suppose you *are* a Marathon Maniac who is planning to run marathons on consecutive weekends, or you have some other reason for wanting to recover as quickly as possible after a race. In that case you will want to skip the pizza and beer and instead practice recovery nutrition by the book. The specific nutrition practices you rely on to bounce back quickly after a race are identical to the ones you should use to promote recovery after workouts throughout the training process, which I alluded to in Chapter 4. These practices may accelerate and heighten the rebound from a race just enough to be worthwhile for high-level runners in certain situations. But when used daily in training the same refueling techniques will make a tremendous difference in the long-term outcomes of the training process for all runners.

What you eat and when you eat after running strongly affect how quickly your body returns to homeostasis, or its normal state of physiological balance. If you consume the right nutrients at the right times the muscle damage you've incurred will heal more quickly, your muscle fuel stores will be replenished faster, and your immune system will rebound more rapidly.

The most important nutrients for immediate postexercise recovery are carbohydrate, protein, water, and antioxidants. Carbohydrate is needed to replenish muscle and liver glycogen stores. Protein is needed to repair damaged muscle cells. Both carbohydrate and protein stimulate the release of insulin, a hormone that facilitates muscle refueling and muscle repair. When carbohydrate and protein are consumed together, muscle glycogen replenishment occurs faster than when carbs are consumed alone and muscle repair proceeds faster than when protein is consumed alone. Carbohydrate and glutamine, an amino acid contained in many proteins, also serve as vital fuels for the immune system and thus aid in the restoration of full immune function after strenuous exertion.

Water is needed after exercise for rehydration, obviously, while antioxidants serve to limit postexercise muscle damage caused by the leaking of free radicals from damaged muscle cells and by the body's own anti-inflammatory response. Sodium and other electrolytes are useful nutrients in a postexercise meal or snack because they are needed to replace the minerals lost through perspiration. They are somewhat less important for immediate postrun recovery than the other nutrients I've identified, however.

Timing is critical. The sooner you take in some carbs, protein, water, and antioxidants, the faster the various recovery processes will unfold. The muscles occupy a unique biochemical state during the first hour or so after a workout or race, a state that enables them to exploit a supply of the right nutrients for recovery far more effectively than they can at a later time. Glycogen replenishment, for example, is achieved 50 percent faster when carbohydrate is consumed immediately after exercise than when it is delayed by several hours.

It's best if the foods you take in immediately after exercise contain little else besides the nutrients that are most helpful to the various recovery processes. Large amounts of fat and fiber, in particular, will retard muscle glycogen replenishment and muscle tissue repair. Liquids are often the best source of immediate postexercise nutrition because the right beverage can provide all of the nutrients needed for recovery in one source and also because it is usually easier to drink than it is to eat in the first hour after strenuous exertion, when appetite tends to be suppressed. Many runners like to drink fruit smoothies with added protein. The dairy industry has lately been pushing low-fat chocolate milk as an excellent recovery beverage, and the research suggests that it is. The milk-enriched tea that Kenyan runners drink so copiously between runs is also a nearly perfect source of nutrition for recovery.

A number of companies make bottled drinks and powdered drink mixes that are formulated especially for nutritional recovery. Although more expensive and somewhat less natural than the options I've identified, the best products in this category are able to provide the precise types and amounts of nutrients that are most effective for recovery while leaving out everything (except colorings and flavorings, in most cases) that does not contribute to recovery or gets in its way.

HOW MUCH?

The optimal amounts of the important postexercise recovery nutrients have been intensively studied. According to this research, 1.2 g of carbs per kilogram of bodyweight are needed to maximize glycogen replenishment after races and workouts that are long enough to severely deplete muscle glycogen stores. This threshold is different for individual runners, but as a general rule I encourage runners to consume 1.2 g of carbs per kilogram they weigh after all runs of 20 miles or more, as well as after all runs of 12 miles or more that include substantial amounts of running in Zone 3 or above. As little as a third of this amount is needed after an easy workout. Studies indicate that roughly 1 g of protein is required for every 4 g of carbohydrate in the first hour after exercise. Certain popular recovery beverages, including Endurox R^4, are formulated to provide the optimal 4:1 ratio of carbs and protein. Continuing to drink by thirst during the first hour after exercise is sufficient to ensure that you rehydrate properly. The optimal types and amounts of antioxidants to consume in the first hour after exercise are not known. A long list of antioxidants, including vitamins C and E (found in tomatoes and spinach, among other foods), flavonoids (citrus fruits), anthocyanins (berries and berry juices), and catechins (tea and dark chocolate), have shown benefits. Very high doses of all antioxidants should be avoided because they are toxic. For example, avoid supplements that provide more than 100 percent of the Daily Recommended Intake of vitamin C or E.

It's probably not a big deal if you wait more than an hour to eat or drink after some of your easier training runs, but I strongly encourage you to make immediate and proper postrun refueling something you do after every run. Recovery and fitness building are closely linked. Many of the physiological adaptations that increase fitness are simply recovery processes that go beyond restoring the body to its prior homeostasis. Because of this the same nutritional practices that help you recover faster from workouts will also help you become fitter in response to training. Powerful proof of this link comes from a study performed by researchers at the University of Texas. In this study thirty-two previously untrained subjects were thrown into an aerobic conditioning program that entailed riding a stationary bike for one hour a day, five days per week for one month. Immediately and one hour after each workout the subjects were given either low-fat chocolate milk (which contains carbs and protein in a ratio close to the 4:1 ideal), a carbohydrate supplement, or a noncaloric placebo drink. (Each subject received the same drink after every session.)

Before the training program started, all of the subjects underwent VO2 max and body composition testing. These tests were repeated after the monthlong training program. Aerobic capacity increased significantly more in the subjects who drank low-fat chocolate milk after each workout. These individuals became fitter in response to precisely the same training that the other two groups did simply because they consumed the right recovery nutrition at the right time. The chocolate-milk drinkers also lost more body fat than those who received the carbohydrate supplement.

Consider each run you do incomplete until you have consumed your recovery nutrition. To ensure that this practice becomes a matter of routine for you, I have included recovery nutrition recommendations in the integrated training and nutrition plans presented in Chapters 10 and 11.

Recovery is affected by more than the nutrition you take in during the first hour after exercise. While this hour is the most important one, your overall diet affects the quality of your recovery more than the postexercise meal or snack alone. In Chapter 1 I explained that consuming the right amount of carbohydrate every day in training will enable your body to better absorb larger workloads. That's because a high-carbohydrate diet helps you recover. A diet that's generally rich in antioxidants will also boost your day-to-day recovery capacity by stimulating adaptive processes, strengthening your immune system, and keeping inflammation in check. Following the guidelines for diet quality balance described in Chapter 2 will ensure that you get enough antioxidants to maximize your recovery in these ways.

THE 8 PERCENT RULE

Most runners gain weight in the first weeks after completing a marathon or half marathon. This is normal, and for many runners it's all but unavoidable. You can't expect to maintain your optimal racing weight year-round any more than you can expect to sustain peak marathon or half-marathon fitness indefinitely. The two go hand in hand. Peak training loads are required to attain maximal leanness. When your training load drops after a big race, your body fat percentage is destined to climb.

Far from a bad sign, postrace weight gain is actually a good sign. Ryan Hall watches the scale carefully to *make sure* he gains 5 to 7 pounds after each marathon because he recognizes weight gain as a measurable sign of his body's regeneration. When the scale registers 135 pounds instead of his racing weight of 130 pounds, Hall knows his body is ready to return to consistent training.

There can be too much of any good thing, though, and postrace weight gain is no exception. While a modest amount of body-fat increase is healthy between training cycles, more than a modest amount is bad. Runners seldom gain so much weight during breaks in their training that their health is affected, but it's not at all uncommon for runners to gain enough weight that it's hard to get back into peak shape and back down to their optimal racing weight for the next big race. Ideally, of course, you would not merely get back where you were previously but build upon the progress you made in your last training cycle. This becomes almost impossible if you really let yourself go between training cycles.

To avoid gaining too much weight after a race it's helpful to impose a weight-gain limit. My 8 Percent Rule states that at no time should a runner's weight ever be more than 8 percent greater than his or her optimal racing weight. (For a refresher on your ideal racing weight, see Chapter 2.) If you heed this rule during breaks in your training you will avoid digging a hole that you can't climb out of in time for your next important event. For example, if your ideal racing weight is 150 pounds, and that's how much you weigh when you complete a marathon or half marathon, be sure that your weight does not climb above (150 + [150 × .08] =) 162 pounds during the downtime you enjoy before you begin formal training for your next major competition.

The 8 percent rule is not a license to gain 10 or 15 pounds from *any* starting point. If you're already above your ideal racing weight when you start an off-season break, your margin will need to be smaller. The 8 percent standard should also be understood as a maximum allowable weight gain for *any* runner, but not *every* runner. Those who are naturally resistant to weight gain should set a lower limit because the only way they could gain 8 percent would be to really let themselves go. Ryan Hall's off-season weight-gain target of 5 to 7 pounds represents an increase of 3.8 to 5.4 percent. Eight percent would be too much for him. He would have to become a complete couch potato and live off fried chicken wings to reach that mark.

Making use of the 8 percent rule requires that you weigh yourself consistently during your off-season breaks. The self-awareness that comes from this habit will itself go a long way toward ensuring that you don't put on too much fat before you start training seriously again. Other measures that you can employ to keep your off-season weight gain in check include limiting the number of low-quality foods you eat, the amount of food you eat, the span of time during which you allow yourself to stray from your normal diet, the magnitude of the decrease in your training load and the duration of your break from intensive training.

Choose the measures that are best for you. Just be sure to avoid the mistake of constraining your break from strict eating and hard training so severely that you don't get the physical and psychological regeneration you need between training cycles. This outcome is no better than slacking off and gaining too much weight. Whereas putting on too much fat will set you back in your efforts to achieve your next goal as a runner, failing to regenerate between training cycles will set you up for physical or mental burnout in the next training cycle.

A QUICK START

When runners get back into formal training after some downtime they commonly have two top priorities: regaining lost fitness and losing the weight they gained during their break. The problem is that it's not possible to maximize fat loss and fitness gains simultaneously. The fastest way to lose weight is to sharply reduce food intake. But a sharp reduction in eating sabotages one's efforts to build fitness quickly because it deprives the body of the fuel it needs to perform optimally in workouts and to recover quickly between workouts.

The incompatibility of eating for weight loss and training for performance was demonstrated in an interesting study conducted by William Lunn of Southern Connecticut University. Lunn recruited thirty-four experienced cyclists and separated them into four groups. One group added high-intensity interval workouts to their training to stimulate rapid improvements in anaerobic power. Members of a second group were required to sharply reduce their calorie intake to stimulate rapid weight loss. A third group added intervals *and* went on a diet, while the members of a control group did neither.

As expected, members of the group that added high-intensity intervals to their training experienced improvements in anaerobic power but did not lose weight. Also as expected, the subjects who dieted lost weight but experienced a much smaller improvement in anaerobic power. These two groups demonstrated equal improvements in their power-to-weight ratio, or the number of watts they could churn out per kilogram of body weight in a thirty-second all-out effort (which is an excellent indicator of race performance potential in cycling). The cyclists in the interval-training group owed most of their 9 percent improvement in power-to-weight ratio to gains in power, while members of the diet group owed most of their 9 percent improvement to weight loss.

Based on these results, you might expect that members of the group that combined interval training with dieting gained power, lost weight, and thereby improved their power-to-weight ratio twice as much as the other two groups. That's not what happened. While the athletes in the diet-plus-intervals group lost as much weight as the dieters had, their power improvements were negligible. Consequently, their average increase in power-to-weight ratio was so small that it did not even attain statistical significance. In other words, statistically, the effect of combining interval training for improved fitness and dieting for weight loss was the same as doing neither.

Why? Lunn and his coauthors speculated that calorie restriction had deprived the members of the diet-plus-intervals group of the energy and nutritional raw materials they needed to adapt to the stress imposed by the introduction of high-intensity intervals into their training. Their stepped-up training and reduced eating worked at cross purposes.

Because fitness development and fat loss cannot peacefully coexist as top priorities, I advise runners who are getting ready to ramp up for their next big race after time off to commit to a brief weight-loss phase before they dive back into intensive training. During this four- to eight-week period—which I call a quick start, because its purpose is to give runners a quick start toward their optimal racing weight— body fat reduction is a clear first priority and fitness improvement is a secondary goal.

THE ELEMENTS OF A QUICK START

The duration of your quick start should be determined by how much weight you need to lose. If you're within 10 pounds of your optimal racing weight, four weeks will suffice. If you're more than 10 but less than 20 pounds over your racing weight, a six-week quick start is preferable. If you have more than 20 pounds to lose, do an eight-week quick start. Regardless of how much weight you need to lose, the point of your quick start is not necessarily to get all the way down to your racing weight before you even start formal training for your next important event. The point, again, is to get a speedy initial launch toward your racing weight. You can shed the remaining excess at a slower rate during the training process itself.

Both your diet and your training within a quick start should differ from your diet and training within a race-focused training cycle in certain key ways that reflect your short-term priorities. During this time your specific diet and training habits need to promote swift fat loss while also getting you ready for the upcoming training cycle. There are two specific dietary changes and three changes to your normal training habits that you will make at the beginning of a quick start.

1. CREATE A MODERATE CALORIE DEFICIT.

As we saw in Chapter 2, during focused training for a marathon or half marathon it is not necessary to count calories, nor is it advisable to consciously eat less for the sake of losing weight. At that time fitness-building is your top priority, which requires that you eat according to your appetite to ensure that your body is supplied with plenty of food energy. Maintaining very high diet quality will suffice to rid your body of excess fat even as you continue to eat as much as you're hungry for.

The situation changes in a quick start. Your top priority during this period is losing weight quickly and to do this you must consciously reduce the amount of food you eat in order to create the calorie deficit without which weight loss is impossible. In principle, the larger your calorie deficit is, the faster you will drop the pounds. But for runners a modest calorie deficit is better than a large one, even in a quick start. While building fitness may not be your top priority at this time, you're still working out and trying to lay a foundation for the race-focused training to come. Eating too little would sabotage these efforts. Also, if your calorie deficit is too large you will lose more muscle and less fat than you would with a moderate calorie deficit.

In the 1980s researchers at Rockefeller University looked at the effect of daily calorie deficits of different sizes on weight loss. As they expected, the fewer calories the subjects consumed, the more weight they lost. What wasn't expected was where the weight loss came from. In individuals who reduced their daily calorie intake by a moderate amount, 91 percent of the weight lost was fat and a mere 9 percent was lean body mass. But in subjects who severely reduced their calorie intake, fat represented 48 percent of the total weight loss and muscle 52 percent. So it appears that larger calorie deficits result in large amounts of muscle loss. For runners, loss of muscle is likely to reduce strength, power, and overall performance.

I suggest a moderate daily calorie deficit of 300 to 500 calories during a quick start. If you're within 10 pounds of your racing weight, 300 calories is sufficient. If you're more than 10 but fewer than 20 pounds above your racing weight, maintain a deficit of 400 calories per day throughout your quick start. If you're more than 20 pounds over your optimal racing weight, aim to consume 500 fewer calories than your body uses each day. Deficits in this range will enable you to lose weight fairly quickly while preserving muscle mass, especially when they are combined with the other quick-start methods.

To determine how many calories you will eat daily in a quick start it is necessary to subtract your chosen deficit from the average number of calories your body will burn daily in the quick start. There are various online tools you can use to create an estimate of the number of calories your body uses daily. Some are better than others. The best ones for athletes allow the user to input detailed information about exercise. One such calculator can be found at nutritiondata.self.com. When you use this tool, enter the average duration and intensity of exercise you intend to do in your quick start. Even though you will train harder than this on some days and not as hard on others (hence you will burn more calories on some days and fewer on others), these fluctuations will balance out over the course of a full week of training, making your calorie burn estimate and your daily calorie deficit accurate.

DAILY CALORIE DEFICIT BY WEIGHT CHART:	
WEIGHT GOAL	CALORIE DEFICIT
Within 10 pounds	300 calories
Between 10 and 20	400 calories
More than 20	500 calories

2. INCREASE YOUR PROTEIN INTAKE.

When you're trying to lose weight it's helpful to combine a calorie deficit with increased protein consumption. There are two benefits of doing so. First, increasing protein intake reduces the spike in hunger that typically comes with eating less. Adding protein to the diet also increases the proportion of total weight loss that comes from body fat and reduces the amount of muscle mass that is lost.

In a 2010 study conducted at the University of Birmingham, England, two groups of athletes cut calories equally to promote weight loss. But one group got 15 percent of its daily calories from protein (which is about normal) while the other group bumped up its protein intake to 35 percent. The 15 percent group lost more total weight, but more than half of that weight was lean body mass. Members of the 35 percent protein group lost just as much fat without losing any muscle.

Other studies have shown that a less extreme 30 percent protein diet is sufficient to reduce hunger and maximize fat loss during periods of caloric restriction. I recommend that you aim to get 30 percent of your total calories from protein during quick starts. Increasing your protein intake to this level will necessitate a commensurate reduction in carbohydrate consumption, but that's not a problem because your training load is relatively low and you are not pursuing maximum performance at this time.

3. LIFT WEIGHTS.

As a runner you should perform some kind of strengthening exercise year-round. Doing so will improve your running economy and reduce your injury risk. Within quick starts you should strength train more than at other times, for two reasons. First, it will give you a more solid musculoskeletal foundation to take into the next training cycle. In addition, much like increased protein intake, a bigger commitment to strength training in your quick starts will help you retain muscle and shed only unwanted body fat.

In a 1988 study at the University of Michigan, obese men who dieted and lifted weights for eight weeks lost 9.45 pounds of fat and gained 1 pound of muscle. Obese men who dieted without lifting weights lost less fat—7.45 pounds—and also lost 2.35 pounds of lean body mass. One diet, two very different sets of outcomes—all depending on whether the diet was complemented by weightlifting.

I encourage runners to perform three weekly full-body functional strength workouts during quick starts. Weightlifting is preferable to other forms of strength training such as calisthenics and yoga because it builds more muscle and thereby promotes more fat loss.

4. DO FASTING WORKOUTS.

In Chapter 4 I distinguished "training high" from "training low." Training high entails consuming carbs during a run for the sake of maximizing performance in the workout. Training low entails withholding carbs during a run to increase the body's fat-burning capacity.

Within a race-focused training cycle it is prudent to make every other week's longest run a "fasting workout" where carbohydrate is withheld. It would be less prudent to "train low" in every long run because you would then miss out on the complementary benefits that come from attaining a higher level of performance through carbohydrate supplementation. But during a quick start I recommend doing a long fasting run once every week. Long runs undertaken at moderate intensity and without carbohydrate intake burn more fat than any other type of run you can do and thus contribute more to your goal of shedding excess body fat. These workouts will also increase your fat-burning capacity and with it your endurance, a benefit that is of secondary importance at this time.

5. DO VERY SHORT, VERY HIGH-INTENSITY INTERVALS.

Your training volume is necessarily lower during a quick start than it is during the race-focused training cycle. You can't maintain maximum training volume year-round or you'll burn out. Obviously, the higher your training volume is, the more calories you burn. So when your training volume is lower, as it is in a quick start, you need to burn calories in alternative ways.

Very short interval sessions are one such alternative. These workouts consist of large numbers of intervals lasting ten to thirty seconds each and performed at or near maximum intensity. High-intensity intervals contribute to fat loss by creating a huge postworkout fat-burning effect. At the same time, high-intensity intervals help prepare the body for later race-focused training by increasing raw speed and power.

A quick start is not the time to do longer intervals, which are more taxing and race specific than short intervals and tend to trigger a fitness peak very quickly when given more than passing attention. But a quick start is a great time to do very short intervals of maximum or near-maximum intensity, for two reasons. First, the resulting gains in raw speed and power will enable you to perform all of your subsequent training at a higher level. Second, you will not be able to focus on speed and power development at any later time, as more race-specific types of training must be prioritized within the training cycle.

Earlier in the chapter I described a study at Southern Connecticut University in which cyclists who either lost weight through dieting or increased their anaerobic power with high-intensity intervals saw improvements in their power-to-weight ratio, while cyclists who dieted and did intervals saw no such improvement. Why, then, am I advising you to maintain a caloric deficit and do high-intensity intervals in a quick start?

The reason is that improving the power-to-weight ratio is not the goal of a quick start. Shedding excess body fat is the primary goal. And guess what? Even though the subjects in William Lunn's study who dieted and added intervals to their training did not significantly improve their power-to-weight ratio, they lost more body fat than did the cyclists who did only one or the other. On average, body fat dropped by 26.4 percent in the diet-plus-intervals group compared to 19.1 percent in the diet group and 1.9 percent in the interval group.

It is important to point out as well that while the subjects who dieted in this study maintained a daily energy deficit of 500 calories, which matches the largest possible deficit in a quick start, these subjects did not consume extra protein as the quick start requires. This extra protein will ensure that you gain speed and power from doing high-intensity intervals despite your energy deficit.

A small amount of high-intensity interval running goes a long way. I advise runners to perform one full interval workout plus a separate workout with a smaller amount of high-intensity running each week throughout the quick start. You should also be aware that sprinting on level ground is very stressful on the muscles and tendons. For this reason I seldom prescribe it. You can get the strength, speed, power, and fat-loss benefits you seek from maximum-intensity running with less chance of injury if you sprint uphill instead. Hill sprints (ten-second efforts) and hill intervals (twenty- to thirty-second efforts) are the two types of interval training I recommend for runners in a quick start.

Here are some examples of hill sprint and hill interval workout formats:

Hill Sprints: Run for forty-five minutes in heart-rate Zones 1 and 2. (Hill sprints should always follow an easy run because an easy run serves as a good warm-up for hill sprints and because you will never do enough hill sprints to make a complete workout of them. You'll find more detailed info on zones in the next chapter.) Next, do a total of eight sprints, ten seconds each, up a moderately steep to steep hill (5 to 10 percent grade). Walk back down the hill to recover after each sprint.

Hill Intervals: Warm up with ten minutes of easy running in Zones 1 and 2 (again, you'll find more info about zones in Chapter 9). Then run twelve thirty-second sprints up a hill with a moderate gradient (4 to 6 percent) at the greatest speed you can sustain through the last interval (Zone 5). Jog slowly back down the hill for recovery. After you've completed the twelve sprints, cool down with ten minutes of easy jogging in Zone 1.

PUTTING IT ALL TOGETHER

There are as many possible quick start training plans as there are marathon and half-marathon training plans. The plan that is best for you will be appropriate to your running background, current fitness level, and goals. One thing that every runner should do in a quick start is distribute the various types of workout that it encompasses in a sensible way. Here's a basic template that you can use in planning your own quick start:

> **MONDAY**—STRENGTH WORKOUT
> **TUESDAY**—EASY RUN + HILL SPRINTS
> **WEDNESDAY**—STRENGTH WORKOUT
> **THURSDAY**—HILL INTERVALS RUN
> **FRIDAY**—STRENGTH WORKOUT
> **SATURDAY**—CYCLING POWER INTERVALS
> **SUNDAY**—FASTING RUN

If you are an experienced and highly fit runner and you want to do some additional running, I suggest you do easy runs on the same days you do your strength workouts.

Your quick start training should obey the principle of progression, just as your normal marathon and half-marathon training do. In other words, your workouts should be quite manageable in the first week of a quick start and then become gradually more challenging in subsequent weeks. If your quick start lasts longer than six weeks you should place a recovery week, in which your training is moderately reduced, in the middle of it.

While the primary objective of a quick start is to induce fat loss, the same workouts that achieve this objective also serve to establish the perfect foundation to build on when you complete the quick start and begin to train for your next race. For example, doing three full-body strength workouts per week will not only improve your body composition but will also iron out strength imbalances in your body and improve the stability of your joints so you're less likely to get injured during your marathon or half-marathon training.

Time your quick starts so that you're able to transition directly into race-focused training after they are completed. What should that training look like? You're about to find out!

PART THREE
NUTRITION-TRAINING SYNERGY

TRAINING
FOR THE WALL

Every runner knows that both nutrition and training affect performance. Most runners think of these two influences as being fundamentally separate, affecting performance individually in different ways. But nutrition and training aren't really separate at all. Your training influences how your diet affects your body. Likewise, your diet influences your training capacity. To maximize your running performance you must ensure that your training and nutrition practices are aligned to serve the same objective. I refer to this concept as nutrition-training synergy.

The major shared objective of the training and nutrition components of marathon and half-marathon preparation is to push back the wall—to give you the ability to sustain a chosen pace through the entire race without losing momentum in the last few miles. We have thoroughly explored the nutrition side of nutrition-training synergy. It's now time to talk about training—specifically, how training can cooperate with nutrition to push back the wall, and the best way to train to ensure that your glycogen stores last all the way to the finish line of your races.

171

Training is capable of pushing back the wall in several different ways. First of all, effective training increases aerobic capacity, or the body's ability to use oxygen to release energy from carbohydrate and fat. The details of how an increase in aerobic capacity improves marathon and half-marathon performance are complex and not fully understood. The general idea is that an increase in aerobic capacity enables a runner to draw on the body's total energy resources at a higher rate, and thus run faster, without hastening glycogen depletion. Elite male runners whose marathon race pace is under 5:00 per mile burn carbohydrate at a higher rate than do middle-of-the-pack runners who run marathons at 10:00 per mile. But thanks to their higher aerobic capacity, elite runners are able to derive more usable energy out of their carbohydrate fuel supplies, so they are no more likely to hit the wall than slower runners despite using more carbohydrate.

Proper training also lowers the total energy cost of running a marathon or half marathon, and it does so in a couple of ways. First, training tends to reduce body weight. A runner weighing 154 pounds burns approximately 2,950 calories during a marathon. If this runner loses 5 pounds he will lower the total energy cost of running a marathon to approximately 2,854 calories, thereby reducing his chances of bonking due to glycogen depletion. A second way that training lowers the total energy cost of running a marathon or half marathon is by improving running economy, or reducing the amount of oxygen and energy that are required to run at any given pace. As running economy increases, the body's fuel stores are able to stretch farther.

Yet another benefit of proper training is an increase in the amount of glycogen the muscles and liver store. Obviously, the more glycogen your body contains, the longer this crucial energy source will last, even if the rate at which it is used doesn't change. After tapering, a trained runner's body stores roughly twice as much glycogen as does a nonrunner's body.

Finally, and not least important, effective training increases the muscles' capacity to burn fat at higher intensities, so that more glycogen is spared when you're running at your goal marathon or half-marathon pace. This effect of training is related to but not completely accounted for by increases in aerobic capacity.

WHAT IS THE BEST TRAINING APPROACH?

The best approach to training for marathons and half marathons is the one that generates the greatest combined gains in aerobic capacity, leanness, running economy, glycogen stores, and fat-burning capacity. A training approach that does all of these things will minimize your chances of hitting the wall in races and maximize the likelihood that you will achieve your goals. There are many possible ways to approach training for marathons and half marathons. Which of them does the best job of pushing back the wall? The short answer to this question is a simple formula: *Run a lot and run slowly most of the time.* This training approach is often referred to as "the Lydiard method" in honor of the legendary Arthur Lydiard.

THE LYDIARD METHOD

As I mentioned in Chapter 5, Arthur Lydiard began to coach runners in his native New Zealand in the 1950s after a period of experimenting on himself with various training methods. In those days most elite distance runners did the majority of their training in the form of short, high-intensity intervals. They did not run a lot, but what running they did was fast. Lydiard played around with the opposite approach, slowing way down and running prodigious distances day in and day out.

After smashing his personal best times in events ranging from the mile to the marathon at the height of his experimentation, when he was in his midthirties, Lydiard became convinced that he had discovered the right way for all runners to train. This conviction was powerfully validated when tiny New Zealand produced three medal-winning runners—all coached by Lydiard—at the 1960 Olympics. Lydiard's new system quickly spread across the globe and has remained the basis of the training approaches used by most elite runners ever since.

SLOW DOWN AND RUN MORE

Running a lot and running slowly most of the time are the basic elements of the Lydiard system. Of these two, running a lot is primary and running slowly most of the time is secondary. High mileage is really the key to the Lydiard method's effectiveness. Running slowly simply *allows* a runner to run a lot.

Running a lot is a powerful way to increase aerobic capacity. It's not hard to understand why. A number of different physiological responses to training are involved in boosting the body's ability to consume oxygen during exercise. The heart grows larger and more powerful, blood volume increases, the muscle cells produce more mitochondria (where aerobic metabolism occurs), and so forth. All of these changes exhibit a "dose-response" relationship to aerobic exercise. In other words, the more exposure your body gets to the aerobic stimulus of running (up to a point, naturally), the more pronounced these physiological changes become and the more your aerobic capacity increases.

High-intensity exercise—or fast running—is, in fact, a more potent trigger for aerobic development than slow running is. But the body cannot tolerate nearly as much fast running as it can slow running. So although fast running is more effective than slow running on a minute-by-minute basis, doing the highest volume of slow running that your body can handle has greater overall potential to increase your aerobic capacity than doing the highest volume of fast running you can handle.

High-mileage training is also the most effective way to shed excess body fat and lose weight. Again, it's easy to understand why. When you run, your metabolic rate is five to ten times greater than it is at rest. This means you burn calories five to ten times faster when you're running than when you're sitting on a couch. The more time you spend running, the more time your body spends at an elevated metabolic rate, the more calories you burn, and the more weight you drop. A runner who runs 20 miles a week burns an extra day's worth of calories each week. But a runner who runs 40 miles a week burns an extra *two* days' worth of calories, and so forth.

The faster you run, the more your metabolic rate increases. This fact might lead you to believe that high-intensity training is the best way to shed excess body fat and lose weight. But remember that the body cannot tolerate nearly as much fast running as it can slow running. Therefore, as with aerobic development, slow running ultimately has the most potential to make you leaner.

Running a lot is likewise the key to maximizing running economy. Every stride you take is an opportunity for your neuromuscular system to practice the skill of running. The more you run, the more practice your neuromuscular system gets and the more economical your stride becomes. Research has revealed a strong correlation between training volume and running economy.

High mileage is the most effective way as well to increase the glycogen storage capacity of the muscles and liver. The primary physiological stimulus for an increase in this storage capacity is depletion of the glycogen stores in training. The more total time you spend running, the more your body is exposed to glycogen depletion and the more its storage capacity is increased. Glycogen depletion also stimulates an increase in the fat-burning capacity of the muscles. The recurrent depletion of glycogen supplies that happens when you run great distances week in and week out forces your body to rely more on fat to keep you going, and through this experience your body becomes a better fat-burning and glycogen-sparing machine.

All of the foregoing science explains why almost all of today's elite distance runners use a version of the Lydiard method, running high mileage and doing most of their running at slower paces. A survey of runners who competed in the 2004 U.S. Olympic Team Trials Men's and Women's Marathons showed that the men ran 89 miles per week on average and the women ran 72 miles. The men did almost three-quarters of their training slower than their marathon race pace and the women did more than two-thirds of their training at slower paces.

Again, the benefit of slower running is not intrinsic to low exercise intensity. The reason well-coached runners do most of their running at slower speeds is not that slow running builds fitness better than fast running. Rather, they run slowly most of the time because doing so allows them to run a lot, and the more runners run (within their personal limitations), the fitter they get.

THE RISKS OF HIGH INTENSITY

High-intensity running is hard on the sympathetic nervous system, which is responsible for managing the body's fight-or-flight response to stressors, including the stress of exercise. Research has shown that while the sympathetic nervous system bounces back quickly from runs undertaken below lactate-threshold intensity (which is the fastest pace a trained runner can sustain for thirty to sixty minutes), there is an exponential jump in how long it takes the sympathetic nervous system to recover from runs performed at lactate-threshold intensity and above. When runners try to do more than a small amount of training at these higher intensities their sympathetic nervous system becomes chronically overactive, so they gain less fitness despite working harder.

The cost of doing too much high-intensity running was demonstrated by a 2007 study involving club-level Spanish runners. A research team led by Jonathan Esteve-Lanao at the University of Madrid separated twelve subjects into two groups and placed them on slightly different training programs for a period of five months. The two groups did the same total amount of running, but one group did 80 percent of its training below lactate-threshold intensity and the remaining 20 percent at and above the lactate threshold, while the other group did only 67 percent of its training below the threshold and the remaining 33 percent at and above lactate-threshold intensity. Both groups performed test races before and after the five-month training period. All of the runners improved, but members of the lower-intensity group improved a full 30 percent more on average than did members of the high-intensity group. Their superior performance occurred not *despite* the fact that they didn't work as hard but *because* they didn't work as hard.

The Lydiard method does reserve a place for high-intensity training, but that place is small. The typical runner who trains by this system does no more than 20 percent of his running at lactate-threshold intensity and above. The reason the Lydiard method includes some fast running instead of none is that fast running improves fitness in ways no amount of slow running can duplicate. For example, researchers have discovered that exposure to lactate—an intermediate product of carbohydrate metabolism that is produced in greater amounts at faster running speeds—causes the muscles to generate new mitochondria, the little "factories" of aerobic metabolism inside muscle cells. A runner who always runs slowly misses out on this important fitness-boosting stimulus.

Because high-intensity running yields so much improvement so quickly, runners are often tempted to do more than a little training at faster speeds, but this is counterproductive in two ways. First, the additional fast running limits the total amount of running the athlete can do. Second, the additional fast running creates a persistent burden of nervous-system fatigue that the runner carries from day to day. This burden prevents the body from fully absorbing and adapting to the hard work that's done and hampers performance in harder workouts, so that the runner gets less benefit from these sessions especially.

HOW MOST RUNNERS TRAIN

Most runners do not train right to minimize the risk of hitting the wall in marathons and half marathons. They simply don't run enough and they also don't do enough slow running.

The average adult runner who classifies himself or herself as "competitive" runs fewer than 35 miles per week. That's not a bad baseline, but it's not enough running to prepare for one's best possible marathon or half marathon (unless it is supplemented with some cross-training—a topic I'll address a bit later). Although few runners can handle the volume of running that elite runners take on, it has been my observation that most nonelite runners could run significantly more than they choose to do.

In addition to not training enough, most runners train too intensely. In 1993 a team of researchers at Arizona State University asked a group of women runners to describe their training. According to these self-reports, these runners averaged three easy runs, one moderate-intensity run, and 1.5 high-intensity runs per week. But data collected from heart-rate monitors that the researchers gave the women to wear through one full week of training told a different story. In reality they did less than half of their training in the low-intensity range, almost half in the moderate-intensity range, and less than 9 percent in the high-intensity range.

All of these runners could attain better results from their training by making two simple changes. First, they need to slow down. Specifically, they should follow the 80/10/10 rule, doing about 80 percent of their weekly running at low intensity, 10 percent at moderate intensity, and 10 percent at high intensity. Second, they should run more—something that slowing down would enable them to do without increased risk of injury or burnout.

I've seen some amazing breakthroughs happen when runners transition from training in the typical way to the Lydiard way. John Heusner, a thirty-eight-year-old corporate vice president in Eastvale, California, achieved a very respectable marathon PR of 3:24:40 at the 2012 Carlsbad Marathon on a training regimen of 35 miles per week. Trouble was, he had aimed for a Boston Marathon qualifying time of under 3:15 in that race and had been on pace to reach his goal for 20 miles before hitting the wall. Afterward John hired a coach, my friend Mario Fraioli, who gradually increased John's average weekly running volume to 55 to 60 miles, with a peak of 70 miles. Mario also reduced the frequency of John's high-intensity runs and encouraged him to slow down considerably in recovery runs. At the 2012 Santa Rosa Marathon John never hit the wall and finished in 3:00:37.

Chances are you could benefit from making similar changes. The training plans presented in Chapters 10 and 11 will help you do that. They adhere to the 80/10/10 rule and they rely on volume more than intensity to stimulate improvement and push back the wall.

BARRIERS TO HIGH MILEAGE

When runners are asked why they don't run more, their two most common answers are, "I don't have time" and "I'm afraid I would get injured." I have more sympathy for the second answer than I do for the first.

Everyone has time to run more. Scientific surveys have revealed that people who exercise regularly do not have any more free time in their daily lives than people who claim to be "too busy" to exercise, and in my experience runners who run a lot are no less busy than are runners who run less. Several years ago I profiled a triathlete named David Morken for ironman.com. David was the founder and CEO of a thriving high-tech business, a husband, and the father of six children, and yet he found the time to train for Ironman triathlons. If David Morken has time, everyone does. It's a matter of priorities. If you really want to run more you will find a way. It's that simple.

Perhaps you simply *prefer* not to run more than you already do. That's fine. Only you can decide where running sits on your list of priorities. That's not my job. My job is to show you how to become a better runner. And it so happens that the surest way to improve for most runners is to run more!

Fear of injuries is a more legitimate reason to avoid running more. Overuse injuries are all too common in running, and as you might expect, research has demonstrated a link between running volume and injury risk. The more you run, the more likely it is that your body will break down. Few runners have bodies that are durable enough to hold together through 120 miles of running per week as many elite runners do. Durability can be increased, however. Nobody starts off being able to run 120 miles per week, or even 50 miles. If you take a patient and cautious approach to the project of increasing your mileage tolerance, you will eventually be able to run substantially more than you do today without getting hurt more.

Also, don't underestimate the effect that slowing down will have on your mileage tolerance. If you think you can't run more, slow down and then think again. Running slower not only makes every stride less stressful on your body, so that your legs can handle a greater number of strides, but it also makes running more pleasant and thus removes a psychological barrier to running more.

Even if you are an especially injury-prone runner like me, you can still practice a high-volume, low-intensity approach to training by incorporating cross-training into your routine. Since passing my fortieth birthday I have been unable to run on consecutive days without breaking down. So I now run just three to four times a week and supplement my running with five or six sessions a week on a bike or ElliptiGO (an outdoor elliptical trainer on wheels). The overall volume of aerobic training that I do is greater than it was when I ran daily (or twice a day) and did not cross-train, and my marathon times are comparable to those I ran when I was ten years younger. The training plans presented in Chapters 10 and 11 include optional cross-training sessions, which I encourage you to take advantage of if fear of injuries is standing in the way of your running more.

MONITORING AND CONTROLLING TRAINING INTENSITY

To practice the Lydiard method effectively you need some means of holding yourself back from running too hard in the 80 percent of your training time that should be spent at lower intensities. The best tool for this purpose is a heart-rate monitor. Pace monitoring is also a helpful way to control training intensity but it is best used in higher-intensity workouts where you're trying to push yourself. Pace is after all a performance variable, and when you're monitoring it there is an instinctive urge to "race the clock." I've been a strong advocate of pace monitoring in the past, but over the years I have observed that many runners find it difficult to use pace to hold themselves back in workouts that are supposed to be easy. Heart rate works better in this regard because heart-rate numbers tend not to seduce runners into going faster than they should.

To train effectively with a heart-rate monitor you first need to determine what low, moderate, and high intensity mean for you individually in heart-rate terms. Each workout you do should have a primary intensity target. That intensity target is defined by a particular heart-rate zone. There are many heart-rate training systems in use and each has its own way of prescribing zones. The system that I've incorporated into the training plans presented in Chapters 10 and 11 is a five-zone system that I developed for PEAR Sports, a company that makes audio-coaching devices for runners.

Some heart-rate training systems use the individual runner's estimated or test-determined maximum heart rate as the basis for calculating custom heart-rate training zones. The problem with these systems is that maximum heart rate (which is determined mainly by a person's size and age) says almost nothing about the heart-rate ranges that are appropriate for an individual runner's training. So instead I

TABLE 9.1 *5-ZONE HEART-RATE TRAINING SYSTEM*

ZONE NUMBER	ZONE NAME	PERCENT OF LACTATE-THRESHOLD HEART RATE
1	Low aerobic	75–80
2	Moderate aerobic	81–89
3	Threshold	96–100
4	VO2 max	102–105
5	Speed	106+

use a runner's test-determined lactate-threshold heart rate as the basis for calculating custom heart-rate training zones. The scientific definition of lactate-threshold heart rate is the heart rate that corresponds to the running intensity at which the muscles begin to produce lactate faster than they can use it. That definition is not particularly important. What's important is knowing your individual lactate-threshold heart rate because some of your workouts should be done at that heart rate and because it can be used to calculate the appropriate intensity for every type of workout you do. Table 9.1 presents my five-zone heart-rate training system.

Zone 1, the low aerobic zone, is a low running intensity that is appropriate for warm-ups and cooldowns, easy recovery runs that are typically done the day after a hard run, and "active recovery" periods between high-intensity intervals.

Zone 2, the moderate aerobic zone, is a moderate running intensity that is appropriate for basic steady-pace runs for aerobic development and long endurance-building runs.

Zone 3, the threshold zone, is a moderately high intensity that corresponds to the fastest pace that trained runners can sustain for thirty to sixty minutes. Training in this zone is a potent means of increasing the capacity to sustain faster speeds for longer periods of time.

Zone 4, the VO2 max zone, is a high but submaximal intensity that encompasses 5K race pace for most runners. The most effective way to train in Zone 4 is to perform multiple Zone 4 intervals of relatively short duration with active recovery periods between them, as this allows you to spend more total time in Zone 4 than you could if you simply ran as long as you could at that pace all in one shot. Training in Zone 4 increases aerobic capacity and the ability to resist fatigue at higher intensities.

Zone 5, the speed zone, ranges from roughly 1-mile race pace to a full sprint. Zone 5 training is always done in interval formats and it's a great way to boost running economy.

HOW TO DETERMINE YOUR LACTATE-THRESHOLD HEART RATE

Step one in the process of determining your personal heart-rate training zones is identifying your lactate-threshold heart rate. The most accurate way to do this is to have a lactate-threshold test done at a professional exercise testing facility. But these tests are expensive, invasive, and inconvenient. Fortunately, there are a couple of field test alternatives to the laboratory tests that are also quite accurate. One is a simple thirty-minute time-trial test. All you have to do is warm up thoroughly and then run as far as you can in thirty minutes (that is, run at the highest speed you can sustain for thirty minutes without slowing) while wearing a heart-rate monitor. Your lactate-threshold heart rate is your average heart rate for the last ten minutes of this time trial. Studies comparing this protocol to lab-based lactate-threshold testing have validated it as extremely accurate.

The only downside of the thirty-minute time-trial field test is that it entails a very stressful, race-level effort that must be repeated once every few weeks to remain current because an individual athlete's lactate-threshold heart rate tends to increase as his or her fitness level does. Lucky for you, there's a second field test that I developed for PEAR Sports that is less stressful yet works just as well. I recently determined my running lactate-threshold heart rate using the PEAR Sports protocol and obtained a value of 160 beats per minute. A few days later I had my running lactate-threshold heart rate determined in a laboratory. The result was 159 bpm. Not too shabby!

The format of this field test is similar to that of the typical laboratory lactate-threshold test. You begin by running at a low intensity and then you incrementally increase your intensity until you reach lactate-threshold intensity. The difference between the laboratory test and mine is that in the laboratory test, each intensity level is quantified by the concentration of lactate in your bloodstream, whereas in the PEAR Sports test each intensity level is quantified by a rating of perceived effort on a basic 1–10 scale. If you own a PEAR Sports device, doing the test couldn't be easier. You just strap on the device, power it up, and follow the voice prompts I give you through the headphones. (There's also a PEAR app for smartphones.) If you don't have a PEAR Sports device, it's still very easy. Follow the steps in Table 9.2.

Once you've obtained your current lactate-threshold heart rate, you can easily calculate your custom heart-rate training zones. Simply multiply your lactate-threshold heart rate by the percentages that define each zone as shown in Table 9.1. Table 9.3 presents an example of heart-rate zones based on a lactate-threshold heart rate of 160 bpm.

If you lack experience in working with perceived exertion ratings, you might need to do the PEAR Sports lactate-threshold test two or three times before you feel fully confident in your ratings and results. What's great about it is that the whole thing takes only twenty minutes to complete and requires that you spend only three minutes at lactate-threshold intensity, which is only a moderately high intensity, so you can easily do it on consecutive days.

Note that heart-rate monitoring is not the best way to monitor and control intensity in Zone 5 because of a phenomenon known as cardiac lag. When you suddenly increase your running pace it may take your heart rate as long as a minute to "catch up" to the higher intensity. Training efforts in Zone 5 are typically short because these intensities are simply too high to be sustained for very long. A typical workout targeting Zone 5 is ten intervals of forty-five seconds in Zone 5 separated by ninety-second recovery jogs in Zone 1. When you do this workout, your heart rate will climb steadily throughout each forty-five-second Zone 5 interval and may never actually reach Zone 5 even though you are running at the right speed—that is, at a speed that *would* elevate your heart rate to Zone 5 eventually. Similarly, your heart rate will fall steadily throughout each recovery jog and may never get all the way down to Zone 1 even though, again, you're running at the right speed.

TABLE 9.2 *PEAR SPORTS LACTATE-THRESHOLD FIELD TEST*

STEP 1	Choose a smooth, flat route for the test and put on your heart-rate monitor.
STEP 2	Start jogging at a very comfortable pace—somewhat slower than you normally like to run. Hold yourself back to a pace that barely seems like exercise.
STEP 3	After 1 minute, start thinking about your perceived exertion level. Adjust it so that you would rate your effort as a 1 on our 1–10 scale, which is described as "very, very easy." You should be supremely comfortable, almost feeling as though you could run all day at this effort.
STEP 4	After 5 minutes increase your effort very slightly from a 1 rating ("very, very easy") to a 2 rating ("very easy"). At this intensity you should still feel as though you're holding yourself back a little.
STEP 5	After 2 minutes at this intensity (or 7 total minutes into the run), increase your effort from a 2 rating ("very easy") to a 3 rating ("easy"). At this intensity level you should no longer feel as though you're holding yourself back but you're still 100 percent comfortable.
STEP 6	After 2 more minutes (or 9 total minutes into the run), increase your effort from a 3 rating ("easy") to a 4 rating ("fairly easy"). At this intensity you feel that you are pushing the pace just a bit but there is no strain whatsoever.
STEP 7	After 2 more minutes (or 11 total minutes into the run), increase your effort from a 4 rating ("fairly easy") to a 5 rating ("very slightly hard"). At this intensity level you must concentrate on making yourself run somewhat fast but you're still totally in control and feeling strong.
STEP 8	After 2 more minutes (or 13 total minutes into the run), increase your effort from a 5 rating ("very slightly hard") to a 6 rating ("somewhat hard"). This is your lactate-threshold intensity. Some runners describe the feeling of running at this intensity as "comfortably hard." You will feel that you are pushing yourself, but you could still keep running at this pace for a while. Your breathing will be deep but controlled.
STEP 9	Sustain this intensity for 3 minutes. If your heart-rate monitor allows you to get your average heart rate for individual "laps" of a run, hit the lap button 2 minutes into this 3-minute segment and again at the end of it to capture your average heart rate. Otherwise just eyeball it. In any case, your average heart rate during that period is your approximate lactate-threshold heart rate.
STEP 10	Complete the run with a 4-minute cooldown at a low intensity. This makes the total duration of the test a nice, round 20 minutes.

Because of cardiac lag I recommend that you use perceived effort to monitor workout efforts that target Zone 5. To do so you must first learn what a Zone 5 effort feels like. All this requires is that you experiment a bit to find the slowest pace that raises your heart rate into your personal Zone 5 range if sustained long enough. Pay close attention to how this effort feels and then recreate that feeling in workouts that call for Zone 5 intervals so that you're able to give a true Zone 5 effort even if the intervals are not long enough to lift your heart rate into Zone 5.

Indeed, it's helpful to get a feel for all five pace zones. This will help you start your efforts in each zone at the right intensity. For example, tempo runs (which I will describe more thoroughly in the next section) feature a prolonged effort in Zone 3 that follows a warm-up in Zones 1 and 2. While tempo efforts always last long enough for the heart rate to climb into Zone 3, there will still be a lag of at least thirty seconds between the start of a Zone 3 tempo effort and the time your heart rate actually reaches Zone 3. If you have a solid sense of the perceived effort that corresponds to your Zone 3 heart rate you will have no trouble starting your tempo efforts at the right intensity even before your heart-rate monitor confirms it.

TYPES OF RUNS

There are three broad categories of runs that every runner should incorporate into his or her marathon and half-marathon training: low- and moderate-intensity runs targeting Zones 1 and 2, moderately high-intensity runs targeting Zone 3, and high-intensity runs targeting Zones 4 and 5. Within each of these general categories are specific types of runs. Let's take a look at the benefits and general structure of each type of workout. I'll also give you a specific example of each type drawn from the training plans in Chapters 10 and 11 and show how to "decode" it so that the plans make sense to you.

LOW- AND MODERATE-INTENSITY RUNS

RECOVERY RUN

Recovery runs are very easy runs that are done entirely in Zone 1. Recovery runs are intended to provide a gentle training stimulus the day

TABLE 9.3 *EXAMPLE OF HEART RATE ZONES FOR AN ATHLETE WITH A LACTATE-THRESHOLD HEART RATE (LT HR) OF 160 BPM*

ZONE	CALCULATION	HEART RATE RANGE
1	LT HR (160) × 0.75–0.80	120–128
2	LT HR (160) × 0.81–0.89	129–142
3	LT HR (160) × 0.96–1.00	153–160
4	LT HR (160) × 1.02–1.05	163–168
5	LT HR (160) × 1.06	169+

after a hard workout, when your body is not fully recovered and thus not yet prepared for more hard work.

Example of a recovery run:

25:00 Z1   Run for 25 minutes at a steady effort level within heart-rate Zone 1.

FOUNDATION RUN

A foundation run is a steady effort of moderate duration in Zone 2 sandwiched between a warm-up and a cooldown in Zone 1. This type of run is the bread and butter of marathon and half-marathon training. You should do more foundation runs than any other type of run. These workouts serve to develop a foundation of aerobic fitness and endurance.

Example of a foundation run:

5:00 Z1   Warm up for 5 minutes in heart-rate Zone 1. Then run for
20:00 Z2   20 minutes at a steady pace within Zone 2. Finally, cool down
5:00 Z1   for 5 minutes back in Zone 1.

LONG RUN

A third major type of workout within the low- to-moderate-intensity run category is the long run. A long run is simply a long foundation run. These workouts serve to increase endurance.

Example of a long run:

1.0 mile Z1   Warm up for 1 mile in heart-rate Zone 1. Then run 7.5 miles
7.5 miles   at a steady pace within Zone 2. Finally, cool down for
0.5 mile Z1   0.5 mile back in Zone 1.

Note that long runs are the only type of run that I prescribe by distance instead of time. The reason is that, for most workouts, time is a better way to give runners of different abilities an equal challenge. For example, if I tell two runners to run 5 miles, and one of them runs ten-minute miles and the other runs six-minute miles, the slower runner is going to be out on the roads for almost an hour, whereas the faster runner is only going to get a half-hour of training. It's better to give everyone a time and let the faster runner cover more distance in that time. But long runs are different, because their job is to build the endurance needed to cover a particular race distance. So long runs really need to be given in distance to provide every runner with equal preparation to go the distance in their races.

MODERATELY HIGH-INTENSITY RUNS

TEMPO RUN

The most commonly practiced type of workout in the moderately-high-intensity category is the tempo run. The typical tempo run consists of a prolonged effort of ten to forty minutes in Zone 3 sandwiched between a warm-up and a cooldown. Tempo runs increase the lactate threshold, or the maximum speed that a runner is able to sustain for thirty to sixty minutes.

Example of a tempo run:

5:00 Z1	Warm up for 5 minutes in heart-rate Zone 1. Then run for 5
5:00 Z2	minutes in Zone 2 to continue getting your body ready for faster
15:00 Z3	running. Next, run for 15 minutes at a steady pace within Zone
5:00 Z2	3. After completing the tempo segment of the workout, run for
5:00 Z1	5 minutes in Zone 2. Finally, cool down for 5 minutes back in
	Zone 1.

FAST-FINISH RUN

A second type of run that targets the middle intensity range is the fast-finish run. A fast-finish run is essentially a foundation run with a relatively short effort in Zone 3 tacked onto the end. Fast-finish runs yield the same benefits as tempo runs do, but they're a little easier.

Example of a fast-finish run:

5:00 Z1	Warm up for 5 minutes in heart-rate Zone 1. Then run for
20:00 Z2	20 minutes at a steady pace within Zone 2. Finally, run for
5:00 Z3	5 minutes in Zone 3.

HIGH-INTENSITY RUNS

The three major types of runs that target Zones 4 and 5 are interval runs, speed-play runs, and hill repetitions. All three are used to increase aerobic capacity and running economy and improve resistance to fatigue at higher intensities. Hill repetitions also build stride-specific strength and power.

INTERVAL RUN

An interval run comprises multiple short efforts at high intensities separated by active recoveries. These runs should be done on a running track or other flat, smooth course conducive to fast running.

Example of an interval run:

5:00 Z1	Warm up for 5 minutes in heart-rate Zone 1. Then run for
5:00 Z2	5 minutes in Zone 2 to continue getting your body ready
5 × (3:00 Z4/2:30 Z1)	for faster running. Next, run for 3 minutes in Zone 4. After
5:00 Z1	you complete this interval, recover for 2.5 minutes in Zone 1. Repeat this interval/recovery sequence four more times. Finally, cool down for 5 minutes back in Zone 1.

HILL REPETITIONS RUN

A hill repetitions run is simply an interval run performed on a hill. Hill repetitions runs yield many of the same benefits as interval runs do, but because they entail work against gravity they build more strength in the legs.

Example of a hill repetitions run:

5:00 Z1	Warm up for 5 minutes in heart-rate Zone 1. Then run for
5:00 Z2	5 minutes in Zone 2 to continue getting your body ready
10 × (1:00 Z5 uphill/	for faster running. Next, run for 1 minute uphill in Zone 5.
2:30 Z1)	After you complete this uphill effort, recover for 2.5 minutes
5:00 Z1	in Zone 1. Repeat this uphill effort/recovery sequence nine more times. Finally, cool down for 5 minutes back in Zone 1.

SPEED-PLAY RUN

A speed-play run is a hybrid between a foundation run and an interval run that is conducted on roads or trails rather than on a track. In a typical speed-play run the high-intensity intervals are shorter (hence less challenging) than in an interval run, but the recovery segments between intervals are done in Zone 2 instead of Zone 1 and are therefore more challenging than the recoveries in an interval run.

Example of a speed-play run:

5:00 Z1	Warm up for 5 minutes in heart-rate Zone 1. Then run for
5:00 Z2	5 minutes in Zone 2 to continue getting your body ready
6 × (0:30 Z5/2:30 Z2)	for faster running. Next, run for 30 seconds in Zone 5.
5:00 Z2	After you complete this speed-play interval, recover for
5:00 Z1	2.5 minutes in Zone 2. Repeat this interval/recovery sequence five more times. When you've completed the full set of speed-play intervals, run for 5 minutes in Zone 2. Finally, cool down for 5 minutes back in Zone 1.

PLANNING YOUR TRAINING

Training for a marathon or half marathon is simply a matter of stringing together the various types of runs in a sensible sequence that builds your running fitness incrementally from its current level to a peak level. The first important decision you need to make when planning your training for a marathon or half marathon is how many weeks to allow yourself to build toward peak fitness. As a general rule, the farther you are from peak fitness when you start training, the more time you need. If you are a beginner or are starting over after a break, you should give yourself at least sixteen weeks to get ready for a half marathon and as many as twenty-four weeks to prepare for a marathon. To devote any more than twenty-four weeks to building fitness for a race is to risk burnout. The human body can only absorb increasing training loads for so long before it needs a break. If you already have a solid base of aerobic fitness, you may need as little as eight weeks of specific training to prepare for a half marathon and ten weeks to get ready for a marathon.

After deciding how long you will train for your next big race, you must next settle on a basic recurring weekly workout structure. Do some form of aerobic workout, preferably running, at least six times per week. Each week, do one longer run, one run that includes a "tempo" effort in Zone 3, and one run that includes efforts in Zone 4 or Zone 5. Here's a sensible recurring weekly schedule to use:

MONDAY: REST, EASY RUN, OR EASY CROSS-TRAINING
TUESDAY: TEMPO RUN
WEDNESDAY: EASY RUN OR EASY CROSS-TRAINING
THURSDAY: EASY RUN OR EASY CROSS-TRAINING
FRIDAY: SPEED RUN
SATURDAY: EASY RUN OR EASY CROSS-TRAINING
SUNDAY: LONG RUN

Throughout most of the process of preparing for a marathon or half marathon, your tempo and speed work should be kept very manageable. For example, on Tuesday you might do a fast-finish run that begins with thirty-five minutes in Zones 1 and 2 and concludes with ten minutes in Zone 3. On Friday you might do a speed-play run that consists of forty-five minutes mostly in Zone 2 with half a dozen thirty-second bursts in Zone 5 sprinkled throughout it.

Beginning eight to six weeks before your marathon or half marathon, you can start to make these weekly higher-intensity efforts a little more challenging. For example, you might build up to doing a tempo run in which you run for thirty minutes in Zone 3. Your hardest speed workout might be a track session consisting of five three-minute efforts in Zone 4 with 2:30 Zone 1 recoveries between intervals.

Do no more than a handful of such workouts to sharpen up for your half marathon or marathon in the final weeks of your program. A little bit of this stuff really goes a long way if you're also doing a lot of slow, comfortable running (or a combination of easy running and cross-training).

As Arthur Lydiard used to say, "Train, don't strain."

NUTRITION-TRAINING PLANS FOR THE HALF MARATHON

CHAPTER 10

Here you will find three sixteen-week integrated training and nutrition plans for the half marathon. The Level 1 plan is for first-timers, the Level 2 plan is for more experienced runners seeking improvement, and the Level 3 plan is for advanced competitive runners. None of these plans is likely to be a perfect fit for you right out of the box, so I encourage you to make small adjustments to further customize whichever plan fits you best. For example, if you would rather rest on Sunday than Monday, go ahead and shift the entire weekly workout schedule back one day. If you'd like to do a 5K race or 10K race as a tune-up along the way (there are no tune-up races baked into the plans), go ahead and insert one, ideally at the end of a recovery week.

All of the running workouts are heart-rate based. Refer to Chapter 9 for guidelines on using my five-zone heart-rate training system. That chapter also provides information on how to perform each type of run included in the training plans.

In addition to the various types of runs, each plan incorporates optional cross-training workouts. I strongly recommend that you exercise

191

this option by doing some form of nonimpact cardiovascular exercise (such as bicycling) to supplement your running. This will increase your aerobic fitness and running performance without increasing your injury risk. It will also help you reach your optimal racing weight and enhance the health benefits of your training. These supplemental workouts should be of moderate intensity and not so long that they interfere with your ability to perform well in your more important runs.

The plans do not include strength workouts, but you should consider these an option as well. Doing just two twenty-minute circuits of bodyweight exercises (push-ups, lunges, etc.) in front of the television a couple of evenings per week will give you meaningful benefits without overdrawing from your energy reserves or overburdening your schedule. If you are ambitious and have the time, you can take a more aggressive approach toward strength training that is closer to the one I recommend for quick start periods in Chapter 8.

On the nutrition side, the plans include daily guidelines for during-workout and postworkout nutrition and weekly guidelines for general diet (except during special periods such as the taper, when the general diet guidelines become daily). Refer to Chapter 5 for more details on nutrition during workouts, to Chapter 8 for further information on postworkout nutrition, to Chapter 1 for a refresher course on daily carbohydrate intake, and to Chapter 5 for everything you need to know about taper nutrition.

The diet-quality aspect of your general training diet is not integrated into these plans, but it is integrated into the training and nutrition journal provided in the appendix. There you will find space to total up how many times you eat each of the ten basic categories of food every week.

If you'd like more personalized coaching, interactive audio versions of the plans are available at pearsports.com. To use them you will need to own a PEAR Sports device such as the Square One. Simply download the workouts onto the device—which includes a heart-rate monitor, a foot pod for speed and distance tracking, a mini computer, and headphones—and follow my verbal instructions as I guide you through each workout and give you tips on diet, injury prevention, motivation, and more.

LEVEL 1 HALF-MARATHON PLAN

This sixteen-week integrated training and nutrition plan for the half marathon is a good fit for runners who are training for their first half marathon or who need or prefer a low-volume approach to training for whatever reason. The schedule prescribes four runs per week plus two optional cross-training workouts. You should be able to comfortably run 4 miles before you start the program.

The hardest week of training is Week 15, which calls for approximately four hours of running including a 12-mile Long Run. Weeks 4, 8, and 12 are reduced-volume recovery weeks. The program ends with a one-week taper.

TABLE 10.1 *LEVEL 1 HALF-MARATHON PLAN*

LEVEL 1 / WEEK 1

	WORKOUT	NUTRITION DURING WORKOUT	RECOVERY NUTRITION (WITHIN 45:00 OF COMPLETING WORKOUT)	GENERAL DIET
M	Rest			3–4 g CHO per kg body weight
T	Foundation run 5:00 Z1 15:00 Z2 5:00 Z1	Water, water + electrolytes, or nothing	At least 0.4 g CHO, 0.1 g PRO per kg body weight	
W	Cross-training Optional			
T	Foundation run 5:00 Z1 15:00 Z2 5:00 Z1	Water, water + electrolytes, or nothing	At least 0.4 g CHO, 0.1 g PRO per kg body weight	
F	Foundation run 5:00 Z1 15:00 Z2 5:00 Z1	Water, water + electrolytes, or nothing	At least 0.4 g CHO, 0.1 g PRO per kg body weight	
S	Cross-training Optional			
S	Long run 0.5 mile Z1 3.0 miles Z2 0.5 mile Z1	Water, water + electrolytes, or nothing	At least 0.4 g CHO, 0.1 g PRO per kg body weight	

LEVEL 1 / WEEK 2

	WORKOUT	NUTRITION DURING WORKOUT	RECOVERY NUTRITION (WITHIN 45:00 OF COMPLETING WORKOUT)	GENERAL DIET
M	Rest			3–4 g CHO per kg body weight
T	Foundation run 5:00 Z1 20:00 Z2 5:00 Z1	Water, water + electrolytes, or nothing	At least 0.4 g CHO, 0.1 g PRO per kg body weight	
W	Cross-training Optional			
T	Foundation run 5:00 Z1 20:00 Z2 5:00 Z1	Water, water + electrolytes, or nothing	At least 0.4 g CHO, 0.1 g PRO per kg body weight	
F	Foundation run 5:00 Z1 20:00 Z2 5:00 Z1	Water, water + electrolytes, or nothing	At least 0.4 g CHO, 0.1 g PRO per kg body weight	
S	Cross-training Optional			
S	Long run 0.5 mile Z1 3.5 miles Z2 0.5 mile Z1	Water, water + electrolytes, or nothing	At least 0.4 g CHO, 0.1 g PRO per kg body weight	

CHO = CARBOHYDRATE
PRO = PROTEIN

		NUTRITION DURING WORKOUT	RECOVERY NUTRITION (WITHIN 45:00 OF COMPLETING WORKOUT)	GENERAL DIET
	LEVEL 1 / WEEK 3			
	WORKOUT			
M	**Rest**			3–4 g CHO per kg body weight
T	**Speed-play run** 5:00 Z1 5:00 Z2 5 × (0:15 Z5/2:45 Z2) 5:00 Z1	Water, water + electrolytes, or nothing	At least 0.4 g CHO, 0.1 g PRO per kg body weight	
W	**Cross-training** Optional			
T	**Foundation run** 5:00 Z1 20:00 Z2 5:00 Z1	Water, water + electrolytes, or nothing	At least 0.4 g CHO, 0.1 g PRO per kg body weight	
F	**Fast-finish run** 5:00 Z1 20:00 Z2 5:00 Z3	Water, water + electrolytes, or nothing	At least 0.4 g CHO, 0.1 g PRO per kg body weight	
S	**Cross-training** Optional			
S	**Long run** 0.5 mile Z1 4.5 miles Z2 0.5 mile Z1	Water, water + electrolytes, or nothing	At least 0.4 g CHO, 0.1 g PRO per kg body weight	

		NUTRITION DURING WORKOUT	RECOVERY NUTRITION (WITHIN 45:00 OF COMPLETING WORKOUT)	GENERAL DIET
	LEVEL 1 / WEEK 4 / RECOVERY WEEK			
	WORKOUT			
M	**Rest**			3–4 g CHO per kg body weight
T	**Speed-play run** 5:00 Z1 5:00 Z2 5 × (0:15 Z5/2:45 Z2) 5:00 Z1	Water, water + electrolytes, or nothing	At least 0.4 g CHO, 0.1 g PRO per kg body weight	
W	**Cross-training** Optional			
T	**Foundation run** 5:00 Z1 20:00 Z2 5:00 Z1	Water, water + electrolytes, or nothing	At least 0.4 g CHO, 0.1 g PRO per kg body weight	
F	**Fast-finish run** 5:00 Z1 20:00 Z2 5:00 Z3	Water, water + electrolytes, or nothing	At least 0.4 g CHO, 0.1 g PRO per kg body weight	
S	**Cross-training** Optional			
S	**Long run** 0.5 mile Z1 3.5 miles Z2 0.5 mile Z1	Water, water + electrolytes, or nothing	At least 0.4 g CHO, 0.1 g PRO per kg body weight	

LEVEL 1 / WEEK 5				
	WORKOUT	NUTRITION DURING WORKOUT	RECOVERY NUTRITION (WITHIN 45:00 OF COMPLETING WORKOUT)	GENERAL DIET
M	Rest			3–4 g CHO per kg body weight
T	Hill repetitions run 5:00 Z1 5:00 Z2 5 × (0:30 Z5/2:30 Z1) 5:00 Z1	Water, water + electrolytes, or nothing	At least 0.4 g CHO, 0.1 g PRO per kg body weight	
W	Cross-training Optional			
T	Foundation run 5:00 Z1 25:00 Z2 5:00 Z1	Water, water + electrolytes, or nothing	At least 0.4 g CHO, 0.1 g PRO per kg body weight	
F	Fast-finish run 5:00 Z1 25:00 Z2 5:00 Z3	Water, water + electrolytes, or nothing	At least 0.4 g CHO, 0.1 g PRO per kg body weight	
S	Cross-training Optional			
S	Long run 0.5 mile Z1 5 miles Z2 0.5 mile Z1	Sports drink or gels + water	At least 0.4 g CHO, 0.1 g PRO per kg body weight	

LEVEL 1 / WEEK 6				
	WORKOUT	NUTRITION DURING WORKOUT	RECOVERY NUTRITION (WITHIN 45:00 OF COMPLETING WORKOUT)	GENERAL DIET
M	Rest			3–4 g CHO per kg body weight
T	Hill repetitions run 5:00 Z1 5:00 Z2 7 × (0:30 Z5/2:30 Z1) 5:00 Z1	Water, water + electrolytes, or nothing	At least 0.6 g CHO, 0.1 g PRO per kg body weight	
W	Cross-training Optional			
T	Foundation run 5:00 Z1 25:00 Z2 5:00 Z1	Water, water + electrolytes, or nothing	At least 0.4 g CHO, 0.1 g PRO per kg body weight	
F	Fast-finish run 5:00 Z1 25:00 Z2 5:00 Z3	Water, water + electrolytes, or nothing	At least 0.4 g CHO, 0.1 g PRO per kg body weight	
S	Cross-training Optional			
S	Long run 0.5 mile Z1 5.5 miles Z2 0.5 mile Z1	Water, water + electrolytes, or nothing	At least 0.4 g CHO, 0.1 g PRO per kg body weight	

LEVEL 1 / WEEK 7			
WORKOUT	**NUTRITION DURING WORKOUT**	**RECOVERY NUTRITION (WITHIN 45:00 OF COMPLETING WORKOUT)**	**GENERAL DIET**
M **Rest**			3–4 g CHO per kg body weight
T **Hill repetitions run** 5:00 Z1 5:00 Z2 5 × (1:00 Z5/2:30 Z1) 5:00 Z1	Water, water + electrolytes, or nothing	At least 0.6 g CHO, 0.1 g PRO per kg body weight	
W **Cross-training** Optional			
T **Foundation run** 5:00 Z1 25:00 Z2 5:00 Z1	Water, water + electrolytes, or nothing	At least 0.4 g CHO, 0.1 g PRO per kg body weight	
F **Fast-finish run** 5:00 Z1 20:00 Z2 10:00 Z3	Water, water + electrolytes, or nothing	At least 0.4 g CHO, 0.1 g PRO per kg body weight	
S **Cross-training** Optional			
S **Long run** 0.5 mile Z1 6.0 miles Z2 0.5 mile Z1	Sports drink or gels + water	At least 0.4 g CHO, 0.1 g PRO per kg body weight	

LEVEL 1 / WEEK 8 / RECOVERY WEEK			
WORKOUT	**NUTRITION DURING WORKOUT**	**RECOVERY NUTRITION (WITHIN 45:00 OF COMPLETING WORKOUT)**	**GENERAL DIET**
M **Rest**			Day 1 of 3-day fat-loading test (optional)
T **Hill repetitions run** 5:00 Z1 5:00 Z2 5 × (0:30 Z5/2:30 Z1) 5:00 Z1	Water, water + electrolytes, or nothing	At least 0.4 g CHO, 0.1 g PRO per kg body weight	Day 2 of 3-day fat-loading test (optional)
W **Cross-training** Optional			Day 3 of 3-day fat-loading test (optional)
T **Foundation run** 5:00 Z1 25:00 Z2 5:00 Z1	Water, water + electrolytes, or nothing	At least 0.4 g CHO, 0.1 g PRO per kg body weight	3–4 g CHO per kg body weight
F **Fast-finish run** 5:00 Z1 25:00 Z2 5:00 Z3	Water, water + electrolytes, or nothing	At least 0.4 g CHO, 0.1 g PRO per kg body weight	
S **Cross-training** Optional			
S **Long run** 0.5 mile Z1 5.0 miles Z2 0.5 mile Z1	Water, water + electrolytes, or nothing	At least 0.4 g CHO, 0.1 g PRO per kg body weight	

	LEVEL 1 / WEEK 9			
	WORKOUT	NUTRITION DURING WORKOUT	RECOVERY NUTRITION (WITHIN 45:00 OF COMPLETING WORKOUT)	GENERAL DIET
M	Rest			3–4 g CHO per kg body weight
T	**Speed-play run** 5:00 Z1 5:00 Z2 6 × (1:00 Z4/2:30 Z1) 5:00 Z1	Water, water + electrolytes, or nothing	At least 0.6 g CHO, 0.15 g PRO per kg body weight	
W	**Cross-training** Optional			
T	**Foundation run** 5:00 Z1 30:00 Z2 5:00 Z1	Water, water + electrolytes, or nothing	At least 0.4 g CHO, 0.1 g PRO per kg body weight	
F	**Fast-finish run** 5:00 Z1 25:00 Z2 10:00 Z3	Water, water + electrolytes, or nothing	At least 0.4 g CHO, 0.15 g PRO per kg body weight	
S	**Cross-training** Optional			
S	**Long run** 0.5 mile Z1 6.0 miles Z2 0.5 mile Z1	Sports drink or gels + water	At least 0.4 g CHO, 0.1 g PRO per kg body weight	

	LEVEL 1 / WEEK 10			
	WORKOUT	NUTRITION DURING WORKOUT	RECOVERY NUTRITION (WITHIN 45:00 OF COMPLETING WORKOUT)	GENERAL DIET
M	Rest			3–4 g CHO per kg body weight
T	**Speed-play run** 5:00 Z1 5:00 Z2 6 × (1:30 Z4/2:30 Z1) 5:00 Z1	Water, water + electrolytes, or nothing	At least 0.6 g CHO, 0.15 g PRO per kg body weight	
W	**Cross-training** Optional			
T	**Foundation run** 5:00 Z1 30:00 Z2 5:00 Z1	Water, water + electrolytes, or nothing	At least 0.4 g CHO, 0.1 g PRO per kg body weight	
F	**Fast-finish run** 5:00 Z1 30:00 Z2 10:00 Z3	Water, water + electrolytes, or nothing	At least 0.6 g CHO, 0.15 g PRO per kg body weight	
S	**Cross-training** Optional			
S	**Long run** 0.5 mile Z1 7.0 miles Z2 0.5 mile Z1	Water, water + electrolytes, or nothing	At least 0.6 g CHO, 0.15 g PRO per kg body weight	

	LEVEL 1 / WEEK 11			
	WORKOUT	NUTRITION DURING WORKOUT	RECOVERY NUTRITION (WITHIN 45:00 OF COMPLETING WORKOUT)	GENERAL DIET
M	**Rest**			4–5 g CHO per kg body weight
T	**Speed-play run** 5:00 Z1 5:00 Z2 6 × (2:00 Z4/2:30 Z1) 5:00 Z1	Water, water + electrolytes, or nothing	At least 0.6 g CHO, 0.15 g PRO per kg body weight	
W	**Cross-training** Optional			
T	**Foundation run** 5:00 Z1 30:00 Z2 5:00 Z1	Water, water + electrolytes, or nothing	At least 0.4 g CHO, 0.1 g PRO per kg body weight	
F	**Fast-finish run** 5:00 Z1 30:00 Z2 12:00 Z3	Water, water + electrolytes, or nothing	At least 0.6 g CHO, 0.15 g PRO per kg body weight	
S	**Cross-training** Optional			
S	**Long run** 0.5 mile Z1 8.0 miles Z2 0.5 mile Z1	Sports drink or gels + water	At least 0.6 g CHO, 0.15 g PRO per kg body weight	

	LEVEL 1 / WEEK 12 / RECOVERY WEEK			
	WORKOUT	NUTRITION DURING WORKOUT	RECOVERY NUTRITION (WITHIN 45:00 OF COMPLETING WORKOUT)	GENERAL DIET
M	**Rest**			3–4 g CHO per kg body weight
T	**Speed-play run** 5:00 Z1 5:00 Z2 6 × (1:00 Z4/2:30 Z1) 5:00 Z1	Water, water + electrolytes, or nothing	At least 0.6 g CHO, 0.15 g PRO per kg body weight	
W	**Cross-training** Optional			
T	**Foundation run** 5:00 Z1 30:00 Z2 5:00 Z1	Water, water + electrolytes, or nothing	At least 0.4 g CHO, 0.1 g PRO per kg body weight	
F	**Fast-finish run** 5:00 Z1 25:00 Z2 10:00 Z3	Water, water + electrolytes, or nothing	At least 0.4 g CHO, 0.1 g PRO per kg body weight	
S	**Cross-training** Optional			
S	**Long run** 0.5 mile Z1 6.0 miles Z2 0.5 mile Z1	Water, water + electrolytes, or nothing	At least 0.4 g CHO, 0.1 g PRO per kg body weight	

LEVEL 1 / WEEK 13				
	WORKOUT	NUTRITION DURING WORKOUT	RECOVERY NUTRITION (WITHIN 45:00 OF COMPLETING WORKOUT)	GENERAL DIET
M	Rest			4–5 g CHO per kg body weight
T	**Speed-play run** 5:00 Z1 5:00 Z2 1:00 Z5 2:00 Z1 2:00 Z4 2:00 Z1 3:00 Z3 2:00 Z1 2:00 Z4 2:00 Z1 1:00 Z5 2:00 Z1 5:00 Z2 5:00 Z1	Water, water + electrolytes, or nothing	At least 0.6 g CHO, 0.15 g PRO per kg body weight	
W	**Cross-training** Optional			
T	**Foundation run** 5:00 Z1 35:00 Z2 5:00 Z1	Water, water + electrolytes, or nothing	At least 0.4 g CHO, 0.15 g PRO per kg body weight	
F	**Tempo run** 5:00 Z1 5:00 Z2 15:00 Z3 5:00 Z2 5:00 Z1	Water, water + electrolytes, or nothing	At least 0.6 g CHO, 0.15 g PRO per kg body weight	
S	**Cross-training** Optional			
S	**Long run** 0.5 mile Z1 9.0 miles Z2 0.5 mile Z1	Sports drink or gels + water	At least 0.6 g CHO, 0.15 g PRO per kg body weight	

LEVEL 1 / WEEK 14				
	WORKOUT	NUTRITION DURING WORKOUT	RECOVERY NUTRITION (WITHIN 45:00 OF COMPLETING WORKOUT)	GENERAL DIET
M	Rest			4–5 g CHO per kg body weight
T	**Speed-play run** 5:00 Z1 5:00 Z2 1:00 Z5 2:00 Z1 2:00 Z4 2:00 Z1 4:00 Z3 2:00 Z1 2:00 Z4 2:00 Z1 1:00 Z5 2:00 Z1 5:00 Z2 5:00 Z1	Water, water + electrolytes, or nothing	At least 0.6 g CHO, 0.15 g PRO per kg body weight	

	LEVEL 1 / WEEK 14 / CONTINUED			
	WORKOUT	NUTRITION DURING WORKOUT	RECOVERY NUTRITION (WITHIN 45:00 OF COMPLETING WORKOUT)	GENERAL DIET
W	**Cross-training** Optional			4–5 g CHO per kg body weight
T	**Foundation run** 5:00 Z1 35:00 Z2 5:00 Z1	Water, water + electrolytes, or nothing	At least 0.4 g CHO, 0.1 g PRO per kg body weight	
F	**Tempo run** 5:00 Z1 5:00 Z2 18:00 Z3 5:00 Z2 5:00 Z1	Water, water + electrolytes, or nothing	At least 0.6 g CHO, 0.15 g PRO per kg body weight	
S	**Cross-training** Optional			
S	**Simulator** 0.5 mile Z1 0.5 mile Z2 13.1 km (8.1 miles) @ half-marathon race pace	Practice race nutrition plan	At least 0.8 g CHO, 0.2 g PRO per kg body weight	

	LEVEL 1 / WEEK 15			
	WORKOUT	NUTRITION DURING WORKOUT	RECOVERY NUTRITION (WITHIN 45:00 OF COMPLETING WORKOUT)	GENERAL DIET
M	**Rest**			Start 10-day fat-loading period (65 percent of calories from fat) (optional)
T	**Speed-play run** 5:00 Z1 5:00 Z2 1:00 Z5 2:00 Z1 2:00 Z4 2:00 Z1 5:00 Z3 2:00 Z1 2:00 Z4 2:00 Z1 1:00 Z5 2:00 Z1 5:00 Z2 5:00 Z1	Water, water + electrolytes, or nothing	At least 0.6 g CHO, 0.1 g PRO per kg body weight	Day 2 of 10-day fat-loading period (65 percent of calories from fat) (optional)
W	**Cross-training** Optional			Day 3 of 10-day fat-loading period (65 percent of calories from fat) (optional)
T	**Foundation run** 5:00 Z1 35:00 Z2 5:00 Z1	Water, water + electrolytes, or nothing	At least 0.4 g CHO, 0.1 g PRO per kg body weight	Day 4 of 10-day fat-loading period (65 percent of calories from fat) (optional)

	WORKOUT	NUTRITION DURING WORKOUT	RECOVERY NUTRITION (WITHIN 45:00 OF COMPLETING WORKOUT)	GENERAL DIET
		**LEVEL 1 / WEEK 15 / CONTINUED**		
F	**Tempo run** 5:00 Z1 5:00 Z2 20:00 Z3 5:00 Z2 5:00 Z1	Water, water + electrolytes, or nothing	At least 0.6 g CHO, 0.1 g PRO per kg body weight	Day 5 of 10-day fat-loading period (65 percent of calories from fat) (optional)
S	**Cross-training** Optional			Day 6 of 10-day fat-loading period (65 percent of calories from fat) (optional)
S	**Long run** 0.5 mile Z1 11.0 miles Z2 0.5 mile Z1	Sports drink or gels + water	At least 0.8 g CHO, 0.1 g PRO per kg body weight	Start 7-day caffeine fast (optional) Day 7 of 10-day fat-loading period (65 percent of calories from fat) (optional)

	WORKOUT	NUTRITION DURING WORKOUT	RECOVERY NUTRITION (WITHIN 45:00 OF COMPLETING WORKOUT)	GENERAL DIET
		LEVEL 1 / WEEK 16 / TAPER PERIOD		
M	Rest			Reduce caloric intake by amount equal to average per-day reduction in calories burned through training in taper period compared to Week 15 Day 8 of 10-day fat-loading period (65 percent of calories from fat) (optional) OR Start 5-day fat-loading period (optional) Day 2 of 7-day caffeine fast (optional)
T	**Speed-play run** 5:00 Z1 5:00 Z2 6 × (0:30 Z4/ 2:30 Z2) 5:00 Z1	Water, water + electrolytes, or nothing	At least 0.4 g CHO, 0.1 g PRO per kg body weight	Day 2 of reduced calorie intake Day 9 of 10-day fat-loading period (65 percent of calories from fat) (optional) OR Day 2 of 5-day fat-loading period (optional) Day 3 of 7-day caffeine fast (optional)

		NUTRITION DURING WORKOUT	RECOVERY NUTRITION (WITHIN 45:00 OF COMPLETING WORKOUT)	GENERAL DIET
	LEVEL 1 / WEEK 16 / TAPER PERIOD / CONTINUED			
	WORKOUT			
W	**Cross-training** Optional			Day 3 of reduced calorie intake Day 10 of 10-day fat-loading period (65 percent of calories from fat) (optional) OR Day 3 of 5-day fat-loading period (optional) Day 4 of 7-day caffeine fast (optional)
T	**Fast-finish run** 5:00 Z1 20:00 Z2 5:00 Z3	Water, water + electrolytes, or nothing	At least 0.4 g CHO, 0.1 g PRO per kg body weight	Day 4 of reduced calorie intake Day 1 of 3-day carbo-loading period (70 percent of calories from CHO) OR Day 4 of 5-day fat-loading period (optional) Day 5 of 7-day caffeine fast (optional)
F	**Cross-training** Optional			Day 5 of reduced calorie intake Day 2 of 3-day carbo-loading period (70 percent of calories from CHO) OR Day 5 of 5-day fat-loading period (optional) Day 6 of 7-day caffeine fast (optional)
S	**Rest**			Day 3 of 3-day carbo-loading period (70 percent of calories from CHO) OR Day 1 of 1-day carbo-loading period (10 g CHO per kg body weight) (optional) Day 7 of 7-day caffeine fast (optional)
S	**Half marathon**	Race nutrition plan	Anything you want!	Prerace nutrition plan

LEVEL 2 HALF-MARATHON PLAN

Use this sixteen-week integrated training and nutrition plan to train for your next half marathon if you're ready to work hard to reach the next level but still want to keep your overall training load and time commitment to running manageable. This Level 2 plan includes five runs per week plus one optional cross-training session. You should already be running at least four times per week and up to 6 miles at a time before you start the program.

The training load peaks in Week 15, which includes a 13-mile Long Run and a total of approximately five hours of running. Weeks 4, 8, and 12 are reduced-volume recovery weeks. The program ends with a one-week taper.

TABLE 10.2 *LEVEL 2 HALF-MARATHON PLAN*

	WORKOUT	NUTRITION DURING WORKOUT	RECOVERY NUTRITION (WITHIN 45:00 OF COMPLETING WORKOUT)	GENERAL DIET
		LEVEL 2 / WEEK 1		
M	Rest			3–4 g CHO per kg body weight
T	Foundation run 5:00 Z1 20:00 Z2 5:00 Z1	Water, water + electrolytes, or nothing	At least 0.4 g CHO, 0.1 g PRO per kg body weight	
W	Foundation run 5:00 Z1 20:00 Z2 5:00 Z1	Water, water + electrolytes, or nothing	At least 0.4 g CHO, 0.1 g PRO per kg body weight	
T	Foundation run 5:00 Z1 20:00 Z2 5:00 Z1	Water, water + electrolytes, or nothing	At least 0.4 g CHO, 0.1 g PRO per kg body weight	
F	Foundation run 5:00 Z1 15:00 Z2 5:00 Z1	Water, water + electrolytes, or nothing	At least 0.4 g CHO, 0.1 g PRO per kg body weight	
S	Cross-training Optional			
S	Long run 0.5 mile Z1 5.0 miles Z2 0.5 mile Z1	Water, water + electrolytes, or nothing	At least 0.4 g CHO, 0.1 g PRO per kg body weight	

	WORKOUT	NUTRITION DURING WORKOUT	RECOVERY NUTRITION (WITHIN 45:00 OF COMPLETING WORKOUT)	GENERAL DIET
			LEVEL 2 / WEEK 2	
M	**Rest**			3–4 g CHO per kg body weight
T	**Foundation run** 5:00 Z1 25:00 Z2 5:00 Z1	Water, water + electrolytes, or nothing	At least 0.4 g CHO, 0.1 g PRO per kg body weight	
W	**Foundation run** 5:00 Z1 20:00 Z2 5:00 Z1	Water, water + electrolytes, or nothing	At least 0.4 g CHO, 0.1 g PRO per kg body weight	
T	**Foundation run** 5:00 Z1 25:00 Z2 5:00 Z1	Water, water + electrolytes, or nothing	At least 0.4 g CHO, 0.1 g PRO per kg body weight	
F	**Foundation run** 5:00 Z1 25:00 Z2 5:00 Z1	Water, water + electrolytes, or nothing	At least 0.4 g CHO, 0.1 g PRO per kg body weight	
S	**Cross-training** Optional			
S	**Long run** 0.5 mile Z1 6.0 miles Z2 0.5 mile Z1	Water, water + electrolytes, or nothing	At least 0.4 g CHO, 0.1 g PRO per kg body weight	

	WORKOUT	NUTRITION DURING WORKOUT	RECOVERY NUTRITION (WITHIN 45:00 OF COMPLETING WORKOUT)	GENERAL DIET
			LEVEL 2 / WEEK 3	
M	**Rest**			3–4 g CHO per kg body weight
T	**Speed-play run** 5:00 Z1 10:00 Z2 6 × (0:15 Z5/ 2:45 Z2) 5:00 Z1	Water, water + electrolytes, or nothing	At least 0.4 g CHO, 0.1 g PRO per kg body weight	
W	**Foundation run** 5:00 Z1 25:00 Z2 5:00 Z1	Water, water + electrolytes, or nothing	At least 0.4 g CHO, 0.1 g PRO per kg body weight	
T	**Foundation run** 5:00 Z1 20:00 Z2 5:00 Z1	Water, water + electrolytes, or nothing	At least 0.4 g CHO, 0.1 g PRO per kg body weight	
F	**Fast-finish run** 5:00 Z1 25:00 Z2 5:00 Z3	Water, water + electrolytes, or nothing	At least 0.4 g CHO, 0.1 g PRO per kg body weight	
S	**Cross-training** Optional			
S	**Long run** 0.5 mile Z1 7.0 miles Z2 0.5 mile Z1	Sports drink or gels + water	At least 0.4 g CHO, 0.1 g PRO per kg body weight	

LEVEL 2 / WEEK 4 / RECOVERY WEEK				
	WORKOUT	**NUTRITION DURING WORKOUT**	**RECOVERY NUTRITION (WITHIN 45:00 OF COMPLETING WORKOUT)**	**GENERAL DIET**
M	Rest			3–4 g CHO per kg body weight
T	**Speed-play run** 5:00 Z1 10:00 Z2 6 × (0:15 Z5/2:45 Z2) 5:00 Z1	Water, water + electrolytes, or nothing	At least 0.4 g CHO, 0.1 g PRO per kg body weight	
W	**Foundation run** 5:00 Z1 20:00 Z2 5:00 Z1	Water, water + electrolytes, or nothing	At least 0.4 g CHO, 0.1 g PRO per kg body weight	
T	**Foundation run** 5:00 Z1 25:00 Z2 5:00 Z1	Water, water + electrolytes, or nothing	At least 0.4 g CHO, 0.1 g PRO per kg body weight	
F	**Fast-finish run** 5:00 Z1 20:00 Z2 5:00 Z3	Water, water + electrolytes, or nothing	At least 0.4 g CHO, 0.1 g PRO per kg body weight	
S	**Cross-training** Optional			
S	**Long run** 0.5 mile Z1 6.0 miles Z2 0.5 mile Z1	Water, water + electrolytes, or nothing	At least 0.4 g CHO, 0.1 g PRO per kg body weight	

LEVEL 2 / WEEK 5				
	WORKOUT	**NUTRITION DURING WORKOUT**	**RECOVERY NUTRITION (WITHIN 45:00 OF COMPLETING WORKOUT)**	**GENERAL DIET**
M	Rest			3–4 g CHO per kg body weight
T	**Hill repetitions run** 5:00 Z1 10:00 Z2 7 × (0:30 Z5/2:30 Z1) 5:00 Z1	Water, water + electrolytes, or nothing	At least 0.6 g CHO, 0.1 g PRO per kg body weight	
W	**Foundation run** 5:00 Z1 30:00 Z2 5:00 Z1	Water, water + electrolytes, or nothing	At least 0.4 g CHO, 0.1 g PRO per kg body weight	
T	**Foundation run** 5:00 Z1 30:00 Z2 5:00 Z1	Water, water + electrolytes, or nothing	At least 0.4 g CHO, 0.1 g PRO per kg body weight	
F	**Fast-finish run** 5:00 Z1 30:00 Z2 5:00 Z3	Water, water + electrolytes, or nothing	At least 0.4 g CHO, 0.1 g PRO per kg body weight	
S	**Cross-training** Optional			
S	**Long run** 0.5 mile Z1 8.0 miles Z2 0.5 mile Z1	Sports drink or gels + water	At least 0.6 g CHO, 0.15 g PRO per kg body weight	

LEVEL 2 / WEEK 6				
	WORKOUT	NUTRITION DURING WORKOUT	RECOVERY NUTRITION (WITHIN 45:00 OF COMPLETING WORKOUT)	GENERAL DIET
M	Rest			3–4 g CHO per kg body weight
T	Hill repetitions run 5:00 Z1 10:00 Z2 9 × (0:30 Z5/2:30 Z1) 5:00 Z1	Water, water + electrolytes, or nothing	At least 0.6 g CHO, 0.15 g PRO per kg body weight	
W	Foundation run 5:00 Z1 30:00 Z2 5:00 Z1	Water, water + electrolytes, or nothing	At least 0.4 g CHO, 0.1 g PRO per kg body weight	
T	Foundation run 5:00 Z1 30:00 Z2 5:00 Z1	Water, water + electrolytes, or nothing	At least 0.4 g CHO, 0.1 g PRO per kg body weight	
F	Fast-finish run 5:00 Z1 35:00 Z2 5:00 Z3	Water, water + electrolytes, or nothing	At least 0.4 g CHO, 0.1 g PRO per kg body weight	
S	Cross-training Optional			
S	Long run 0.5 mile Z1 9.0 miles Z2 0.5 mile Z1	Water, water + electrolytes, or nothing	At least 0.6 g CHO, 0.15 g PRO per kg body weight	

LEVEL 2 / WEEK 7				
	WORKOUT	NUTRITION DURING WORKOUT	RECOVERY NUTRITION (WITHIN 45:00 OF COMPLETING WORKOUT)	GENERAL DIET
M	Rest			3–4 g CHO per kg body weight
T	Hill repetitions run 5:00 Z1 10:00 Z2 7 × (1:00 Z5/2:30 Z1) 5:00 Z1	Water, water + electrolytes, or nothing	At least 0.6 g CHO, 0.15 g PRO per kg body weight	
W	Foundation run 5:00 Z1 30:00 Z2 5:00 Z1	Water, water + electrolytes, or nothing	At least 0.4 g CHO, 0.1 g PRO per kg body weight	
T	Foundation run 5:00 Z1 30:00 Z2 5:00 Z1	Water, water + electrolytes, or nothing	At least 0.4 g CHO, 0.1 g PRO per kg body weight	
F	Fast-finish run 5:00 Z1 25:00 Z2 10:00 Z3	Water, water + electrolytes, or nothing	At least 0.6 g CHO, 0.15 g PRO per kg body weight	
S	Cross-training Optional			
S	Long run 0.5 mile Z1 10.0 miles Z2 0.5 mile Z1	Sports drink or gels + water	At least 0.6 g CHO, 0.15 g PRO per kg body weight	

LEVEL 2 / WEEK 8 / RECOVERY WEEK

	WORKOUT	NUTRITION DURING WORKOUT	RECOVERY NUTRITION (WITHIN 45:00 OF COMPLETING WORKOUT)	GENERAL DIET
M	Rest			Day 1 of 3-day fat-loading test (optional)
T	Hill repetitions run 5:00 Z1 10:00 Z2 8 × (0:30 Z5/2:30 Z1) 5:00 Z1	Water, water + electrolytes, or nothing	At least 0.6 g CHO, 0.15 g PRO per kg body weight	Day 2 of 3-day fat-loading test (optional)
W	Foundation run 5:00 Z1 25:00 Z2 5:00 Z1	Water, water + electrolytes, or nothing	At least 0.4 g CHO, 0.1 g PRO per kg body weight	Day 3 of 3-day fat-loading test (optional)
T	Foundation run 5:00 Z1 25:00 Z2 5:00 Z1	Water, water + electrolytes, or nothing	At least 0.4 g CHO, 0.1 g PRO per kg body weight	3–4 g CHO per kg body weight
F	Fast-finish run 5:00 Z1 30:00 Z2 5:00 Z3	Water, water + electrolytes, or nothing	At least 0.4 g CHO, 0.1 g PRO per kg body weight	
S	Cross-training Optional			
S	Long run 0.5 mile Z1 8.0 miles Z2 0.5 mile Z1	Water, water + electrolytes, or nothing	At least 0.6 g CHO, 0.15 g PRO per kg body weight	

LEVEL 2 / WEEK 9

	WORKOUT	NUTRITION DURING WORKOUT	RECOVERY NUTRITION (WITHIN 45:00 OF COMPLETING WORKOUT)	GENERAL DIET
M	Rest			3–4 g CHO per kg body weight
T	Interval run 5:00 Z1 5:00 Z2 6 × (2:00 Z4/2:30 Z1) 5:00 Z1	Water, water + electrolytes, or nothing	At least 0.6 g CHO, 0.15 g PRO per kg body weight	
W	Recovery run 40:00 Z1	Water, water + electrolytes, or nothing	At least 0.4 g CHO, 0.1 g PRO per kg body weight	
T	Foundation run 5:00 Z1 35:00 Z2 5:00 Z1	Water, water + electrolytes, or nothing	At least 0.4 g CHO, 0.1 g PRO per kg body weight	
F	Fast-finish run 5:00 Z1 30:00 Z2 10:00 Z3	Water, water + electrolytes, or nothing	At least 0.6 g CHO, 0.15 g PRO per kg body weight	
S	Cross-training Optional			
S	Long run 0.5 mile Z1 11.0 miles Z2 0.5 mile Z1	Sports drink or gels + water	At least 0.8 g CHO, 0.2 g PRO per kg body weight	

	LEVEL 2 / WEEK 10			
	WORKOUT	NUTRITION DURING WORKOUT	RECOVERY NUTRITION (WITHIN 45:00 OF COMPLETING WORKOUT)	GENERAL DIET
M	**Rest**			4–5 g CHO per kg body weight
T	**Interval run** 5:00 Z1 5:00 Z2 8 × (2:00 Z4/2:30 Z1) 5:00 Z1	Water, water + electrolytes, or nothing	At least 0.8 g CHO, 0.2 g PRO per kg body weight	
W	**Recovery run** 40:00 Z1	Water, water + electrolytes, or nothing	At least 0.4 g CHO, 0.1 g PRO per kg body weight	
T	**Foundation run** 5:00 Z1 35:00 Z2 5:00 Z1	Water, water + electrolytes, or nothing	At least 0.4 g CHO, 0.1 g PRO per kg body weight	
F	**Fast-finish run** 5:00 Z1 35:00 Z2 12:00 Z3	Water, water + electrolytes, or nothing	At least 0.6 g CHO, 0.15 g PRO per kg body weight	
S	**Cross-training** Optional			
S	**Long run** 0.5 mile Z1 12.0 miles Z2 0.5 mile Z1	Water, water + electrolytes, or nothing	At least 0.8 g CHO, 0.2 g PRO per kg body weight	

	LEVEL 2 / WEEK 11			
	WORKOUT	NUTRITION DURING WORKOUT	RECOVERY NUTRITION (WITHIN 45:00 OF COMPLETING WORKOUT)	GENERAL DIET
M	**Rest**			4–5 g CHO per kg body weight
T	**Interval run** 5:00 Z1 10:00 Z2 5 × (3:00 Z4/2:30 Z1) 5:00 Z1	Water, water + electrolytes, or nothing	At least 0.6 g CHO, 0.15 g PRO per kg body weight	
W	**Recovery run** 40:00 Z1	Water, water + electrolytes, or nothing	At least 0.4 g CHO, 0.1 g PRO per kg body weight	
T	**Foundation run** 5:00 Z1 35:00 Z2 5:00 Z1	Water, water + electrolytes, or nothing	At least 0.4 g CHO, 0.1 g PRO per kg body weight	
F	**Tempo run** 5:00 Z1 10:00 Z2 15:00 Z3 10:00 Z2 5:00 Z1	Water, water + electrolytes, or nothing	At least 0.6 g CHO, 0.15 g PRO per kg body weight	
S	**Cross-training** Optional			
S	**Long run** 0.5 mile Z1 13.0 miles Z2 0.5 mile Z1	Sports drink or gels + water	At least 0.8 g CHO, 0.2 g PRO per kg body weight	

LEVEL 2 / WEEK 12 / RECOVERY WEEK				
	WORKOUT	NUTRITION DURING WORKOUT	RECOVERY NUTRITION (WITHIN 45:00 OF COMPLETING WORKOUT)	GENERAL DIET
M	**Rest**			4–5 g CHO per kg body weight
T	**Speed-play run** 5:00 Z1 10:00 Z2 8 × (0:30 Z5/2:30 Z1) 5:00 Z1	Water, water + electrolytes, or nothing	At least 0.6 g CHO, 0.15 g PRO per kg body weight	
W	**Recovery run** 40:00 Z1	Water, water + electrolytes, or nothing	At least 0.4 g CHO, 0.1 g PRO per kg body weight	
T	**Foundation run** 5:00 Z1 30:00 Z2 5:00 Z1	Water, water + electrolytes, or nothing	At least 0.4 g CHO, 0.1 g PRO per kg body weight	
F	**Fast-finish run** 5:00 Z1 25:00 Z2 12:00 Z3	Water, water + electrolytes, or nothing	At least 0.4 g CHO, 0.1 g PRO per kg body weight	
S	**Cross-training** Optional			
S	**Long run** 0.5 mile Z1 9.0 miles Z2 0.5 mile Z1	Water, water + electrolytes, or nothing	At least 0.6 g CHO, 0.15 g PRO per kg body weight	

LEVEL 2 / WEEK 13				
	WORKOUT	NUTRITION DURING WORKOUT	RECOVERY NUTRITION (WITHIN 45:00 OF COMPLETING WORKOUT)	GENERAL DIET
M	**Rest**			4–5 g CHO per kg body weight
T	**Interval run** 5:00 Z1 10:00 Z2 4 × (4:00 Z4/2:30 Z1) 5:00 Z1	Water, water + electrolytes, or nothing	At least 0.6 g CHO, 0.15 g PRO per kg body weight	
W	**Recovery run** 45:00 Z1	Water, water + electrolytes, or nothing	At least 0.4 g CHO, 0.1 g PRO per kg body weight	
T	**Foundation run** 5:00 Z1 35:00 Z2 5:00 Z1	Water, water + electrolytes, or nothing	At least 0.4 g CHO, 0.15 g PRO per kg body weight	
F	**Tempo run** 5:00 Z1 10:00 Z2 20:00 Z3 10:00 Z2 5:00 Z1	Water, water + electrolytes, or nothing	At least 0.8 g CHO, 0.2 g PRO per kg body weight	
S	**Cross-training** Optional			
S	**Long run** 0.5 mile Z1 13.0 miles Z2 0.5 mile Z1	Sports drink or gels + water	At least 0.8 g CHO, 0.2 g PRO per kg body weight	

	WORKOUT	NUTRITION DURING WORKOUT	RECOVERY NUTRITION (WITHIN 45:00 OF COMPLETING WORKOUT)	GENERAL DIET
M	**Rest**			4–5 g CHO per kg body weight
T	**Speed-play run** 5:00 Z1 5:00 Z2 2 × (1:00 Z5/2:00 Z1) 2:00 Z4 2:00 Z1 4:00 Z3 2:00 Z1 2:00 Z4 2:00 Z1 2 × (1:00 Z5/2:00 Z1) 5:00 Z2 5:00 Z1	Water, water + electrolytes, or nothing	At least 0.6 g CHO, 0.15 g PRO per kg body weight	
W	**Recovery run** 45:00 Z1	Water, water + electrolytes, or nothing	At least 0.4 g CHO, 0.1 g PRO per kg body weight	
T	**Foundation run** 5:00 Z1 35:00 Z2 5:00 Z1	Water, water + electrolytes, or nothing	At least 0.4 g CHO, 0.1 g PRO per kg body weight	
F	**Tempo run** 5:00 Z1 8:00 Z2 24:00 Z3 8:00 Z2 5:00 Z1	Water, water + electrolytes, or nothing	At least 0.8 g CHO, 0.2 g PRO per kg body weight	
S	**Cross-training** Optional			
S	**Simulator** 0.5 mile Z1 0.5 mile Z2 13.1 km (8.1 miles) @ half-marathon race pace	Practice race nutrition plan	At least 0.8 g CHO, 0.2 g PRO per kg body weight	

LEVEL 2 / WEEK 14

		NUTRITION DURING WORKOUT	RECOVERY NUTRITION (WITHIN 45:00 OF COMPLETING WORKOUT)	GENERAL DIET
	LEVEL 2 / WEEK 15			
	WORKOUT			
M	Rest			Start 10-day fat-loading period (65 percent of calories from fat) (optional)
T	**Interval run** 5:00 Z1 5:00 Z2 2 × (1:00 Z5/ 2:00 Z1) 2:00 Z4 2:00 Z1 5:00 Z3 2:00 Z1 2:00 Z4 2:00 Z1 2 × (1:00 Z5/ 2:00 Z1) 5:00 Z2 5:00 Z1	Water, water + electrolytes, or nothing		Day 2 of 10-day fat-loading period (65 percent of calories from fat) (optional)
W	**Recovery run** 45:00 Z1	Water, water + electrolytes, or nothing	At least 0.4 g CHO, 0.1 g PRO per kg body weight	Day 3 of 10-day fat-loading period (65 percent of calories from fat) (optional)
T	**Foundation run** 5:00 Z1 35:00 Z2 5:00 Z1	Water, water + electrolytes, or nothing	At least 0.4 g CHO, 0.1 g PRO per kg body weight	Day 4 of 10-day fat-loading period (65 percent of calories from fat) (optional)
F	**Tempo run** 5:00 Z1 6:00 Z2 28:00 Z3 6:00 Z2 5:00 Z1	Water, water + electrolytes, or nothing	At least 0.8 g CHO, 0.2 g PRO per kg body weight	Day 5 of 10-day fat-loading period (65 percent of calories from fat) (optional)
S	**Cross-training** Optional			Day 6 of 10-day fat-loading period (65 percent of calories from fat) (optional)
S	**Long run with fast finish** 0.5 mile Z1 11.5 miles Z2 1 mile Z3	Sports drink or gels + water	At least 0.8 g CHO, 0.2 g PRO per kg body weight	Start 7-day caffeine fast (optional) Day 7 of 10-day fat-loading period (65 percent of calories from fat) (optional)

	WORKOUT	NUTRITION DURING WORKOUT	RECOVERY NUTRITION (WITHIN 45:00 OF COMPLETING WORKOUT)	GENERAL DIET
M	**Rest**			Reduce caloric intake by amount equal to average per-day reduction in calories burned through training in taper period compared to week15 Day 8 of 10-day fat-loading period (65 percent of calories from fat) (optional) OR Start 5-day fat-loading period (optional) Day 2 of 7-day caffeine fast (optional)
T	**Speed-play run** 5:00 Z1 10:00 Z2 8 × (0:30 Z4/ 2:30 Z2) 5:00 Z1	Water, water + electrolytes, or nothing	At least 0.4 g CHO, 0.1 g PRO per kg body weight	Day 2 of reduced calorie intake Day 9 of 10-day fat-loading period (65 percent of calories from fat) (optional) OR Day 2 of 5-day fat-loading period (optional) Day 3 of 7-day caffeine fast (optional)
W	**Recovery run** 45:00 Z1	Water, water + electrolytes, or nothing	At least 0.4 g CHO, 0.1 g PRO per kg body weight	Day 3 of reduced calorie intake Day 10 of 10-day fat-loading period (65 percent of calories from fat) (optional) OR Day 3 of 5-day fat-loading period (optional) Day 4 of 7-day caffeine fast (optional)

LEVEL 2 / WEEK 16 / TAPER PERIOD

	WORKOUT	NUTRITION DURING WORKOUT	RECOVERY NUTRITION (WITHIN 45:00 OF COMPLETING WORKOUT)	GENERAL DIET
			LEVEL 2 / WEEK 16 / TAPER PERIOD / CONTINUED	
T	**Fast-finish run** 5:00 Z1 20:00 Z2 5:00 Z3	Water, water + electrolytes, or nothing	At least 0.4 g CHO, 0.1 g PRO per kg body weight	Day 4 of reduced calorie intake Day 1 of 3-day carbo-loading period (70 percent of calories from CHO) OR Day 4 of 5-day fat-loading period (optional) Day 5 of 7-day caffeine fast (optional)
F	**Cross-training** Optional			Day 5 of reduced calorie intake Day 2 of 3-day carbo-loading period (70 percent of calories from CHO) OR Day 5 of 5-day fat-loading period (optional) Day 6 of 7-day caffeine fast (optional)
S	**Speed-play run** 5:00 Z1 5:00 Z2 4 × (0:30 Z4/ 1:30 Z2) 5:00 Z1	Water, water + electrolytes, or nothing	At least 0.4 g CHO, 0.1 g PRO per kg body weight	Day 3 of 3-day carbo-loading period (70 percent of calories from CHO) OR Day 1 of 1-day carbo-loading period (10 g CHO per kg body weight) (optional) Day 7 of 7-day caffeine fast (optional)
S	**Half marathon**	Race nutrition plan	Anything you want!	Prerace nutrition plan

LEVEL 3 HALF-MARATHON PLAN

The workload in this sixteen-week integrated training and nutrition plan is about as heavy as any runner preparing for a half marathon can sensibly take on without training twice a day. It includes either seven runs or, optionally, six runs and one cross-training session per week in most weeks. You should already be running more or less daily and able to comfortably go at least 7 miles before you start the program.

The most challenging week of the program is Week 14, which includes a half-marathon Simulator (13.1 km at half-marathon race pace) and a total of approximately seven and a half hours of running. Weeks 3, 6, 9, and 12 are reduced-volume recovery weeks. There is a two-week taper starting at Week 15.

	WORKOUT	NUTRITION DURING WORKOUT	RECOVERY NUTRITION (WITHIN 45:00 OF COMPLETING WORKOUT)	GENERAL DIET
	TABLE 10.3 *LEVEL 3 HALF-MARATHON PLAN*			
	LEVEL 3 / WEEK 1			
M	**Foundation run** 5:00 Z1 30:00 Z2 5:00 Z1 OR Cross-training	Water, water + electrolytes, or nothing	At least 0.4 g CHO, 0.1 g PRO per kg body weight	4–5 g CHO per kg body weight
T	**Foundation run** 5:00 Z1 30:00 Z2 5:00 Z1	Water, water + electrolytes, or nothing	At least 0.4 g CHO, 0.1 g PRO per kg body weight	
W	**Foundation run** 5:00 Z1 30:00 Z2 5:00 Z1	Water, water + electrolytes, or nothing	At least 0.4 g CHO, 0.1 g PRO per kg body weight	
T	**Foundation run** 5:00 Z1 30:00 Z2 5:00 Z1	Water, water + electrolytes, or nothing	At least 0.4 g CHO, 0.1 g PRO per kg body weight	
F	**Foundation run** 5:00 Z1 30:00 Z2 5:00 Z1	Water, water + electrolytes, or nothing	At least 0.4 g CHO, 0.1 g PRO per kg body weight	
S	**Foundation run** 5:00 Z1 30:00 Z2 5:00 Z1	Water, water + electrolytes, or nothing	At least 0.4 g CHO, 0.1 g PRO per kg body weight	
S	**Long run** 0.5 mile Z1 6.0 miles Z2 0.5 mile Z1	Water, water + electrolytes, or nothing	At least 0.4 g CHO, 0.1 g PRO per kg body weight	

LEVEL 3 / WEEK 2

	WORKOUT	NUTRITION DURING WORKOUT	RECOVERY NUTRITION (WITHIN 45:00 OF COMPLETING WORKOUT)	GENERAL DIET
M	**Foundation run** 5:00 Z1 35:00 Z2 5:00 Z1 OR Cross-training	Water, water + electrolytes, or nothing	At least 0.4 g CHO, 0.1 g PRO per kg body weight	4–5 g CHO per kg body weight
T	**Speed-play run** 5:00 Z1 10:00 Z2 8 × (0:15 Z5/2:45 Z2) 5:00 Z1	Water, water + electrolytes, or nothing	At least 0.4 g CHO, 0.1 g PRO per kg body weight	
W	**Foundation run** 5:00 Z1 35:00 Z2 5:00 Z1	Water, water + electrolytes, or nothing	At least 0.4 g CHO, 0.1 g PRO per kg body weight	
T	**Foundation run** 5:00 Z1 35:00 Z2 5:00 Z1	Water, water + electrolytes, or nothing	At least 0.4 g CHO, 0.1 g PRO per kg body weight	
F	**Foundation run** 5:00 Z1 35:00 Z2 5:00 Z1	Water, water + electrolytes, or nothing	At least 0.4 g CHO, 0.1 g PRO per kg body weight	
S	**Foundation run** 5:00 Z1 35:00 Z2 5:00 Z1	Water, water + electrolytes, or nothing	At least 0.4 g CHO, 0.1 g PRO per kg body weight	
S	**Long run** 0.5 mile Z1 8.0 miles Z2 0.5 mile Z1	Water, water + electrolytes, or nothing	At least 0.6 g CHO, 0.15 g PRO per kg body weight	

LEVEL 3 / WEEK 3 / RECOVERY WEEK

	WORKOUT	NUTRITION DURING WORKOUT	RECOVERY NUTRITION (WITHIN 45:00 OF COMPLETING WORKOUT)	GENERAL DIET
M	**Rest**			4–5 g CHO per kg body weight
T	**Speed-play run** 5:00 Z1 10:00 Z2 6 × (0:15 Z5/2:45 Z2) 5:00 Z1	Water, water + electrolytes, or nothing	At least 0.4 g CHO, 0.1 g PRO per kg body weight	
W	**Recovery run** 45:00 Z1	Water, water + electrolytes, or nothing	At least 0.4 g CHO, 0.1 g PRO per kg body weight	
T	**Foundation run** 5:00 Z1 35:00 Z2 5:00 Z1	Water, water + electrolytes, or nothing	At least 0.4 g CHO, 0.1 g PRO per kg body weight	

LEVEL 3 / WEEK 3 / RECOVERY WEEK / CONTINUED

	WORKOUT	NUTRITION DURING WORKOUT	RECOVERY NUTRITION (WITHIN 45:00 OF COMPLETING WORKOUT)	GENERAL DIET
F	**Fast-finish run** 5:00 Z1 35:00 Z2 5:00 Z3	Water, water + electrolytes, or nothing	At least 0.4 g CHO, 0.1 g PRO per kg body weight	4–5 g CHO per kg body weight
S	**Foundation run** 5:00 Z1 35:00 Z2 5:00 Z1	Water, water + electrolytes, or nothing	At least 0.4 g CHO, 0.1 g PRO per kg body weight	
S	**Long run** 0.5 mile Z1 7.0 miles Z2 0.5 mile Z1	Sports drink or gels + water	At least 0.6 g CHO, 0.15 g PRO per kg body weight	

LEVEL 3 / WEEK 4

	WORKOUT	NUTRITION DURING WORKOUT	RECOVERY NUTRITION (WITHIN 45:00 OF COMPLETING WORKOUT)	GENERAL DIET
M	**Foundation run** 5:00 Z1 40:00 Z2 5:00 Z1 OR Cross-training	Water, water + electrolytes, or nothing	At least 0.4 g CHO, 0.1 g PRO per kg body weight	4–5 g CHO per kg body weight
T	**Speed-play run** 5:00 Z1 10:00 Z2 8 × (0:30 Z5/2:30 Z2) 5:00 Z1	Water, water + electrolytes, or nothing	At least 0.4 g CHO, 0.1 g PRO per kg body weight	
W	**Foundation run** 5:00 Z1 40:00 Z2 5:00 Z1	Water, water + electrolytes, or nothing	At least 0.4 g CHO, 0.1 g PRO per kg body weight	
T	**Foundation run** 5:00 Z1 40:00 Z2 5:00 Z1	Water, water + electrolytes, or nothing	At least 0.4 g CHO, 0.1 g PRO per kg body weight	
F	**Fast-finish run** 5:00 Z1 40:00 Z2 5:00 Z3	Water, water + electrolytes, or nothing	At least 0.6 g CHO, 0.15 g PRO per kg body weight	
S	**Foundation run** 5:00 Z1 40:00 Z2 5:00 Z1	Water, water + electrolytes, or nothing	At least 0.4 g CHO, 0.1 g PRO per kg body weight	
S	**Long run** 0.5 mile Z1 9.0 miles Z2 0.5 mile Z1	Water, water + electrolytes, or nothing	At least 0.6 g CHO, 0.15 g PRO per kg body weight	

		LEVEL 3 / WEEK 5		
	WORKOUT	NUTRITION DURING WORKOUT	RECOVERY NUTRITION (WITHIN 45:00 OF COMPLETING WORKOUT)	GENERAL DIET
M	**Foundation run** 5:00 Z1 40:00 Z2 5:00 Z1 OR Cross-training	Water, water + electrolytes, or nothing	At least 0.4 g CHO, 0.1 g PRO per kg body weight	4–5 g CHO per kg body weight
T	**Hill repetitions run** 5:00 Z1 10:00 Z2 10 × (0:30 Z5/2:30 Z1) 5:00 Z1	Water, water + electrolytes, or nothing	At least 0.8 g CHO, 0.2 g PRO per kg body weight	
W	**Recovery run** 45:00 Z1	Water, water + electrolytes, or nothing	At least 0.4 g CHO, 0.1 g PRO per kg body weight	
T	**Foundation run** 5:00 Z1 40:00 Z2 5:00 Z1	Water, water + electrolytes, or nothing	At least 0.4 g CHO, 0.1 g PRO per kg body weight	
F	**Fast-finish run** 5:00 Z1 40:00 Z2 5:00 Z3	Water, water + electrolytes, or nothing	At least 0.6 g CHO, 0.15 g PRO per kg body weight	
S	**Foundation run** 5:00 Z1 40:00 Z2 5:00 Z1	Water, water + electrolytes, or nothing	At least 0.4 g CHO, 0.1 g PRO per kg body weight	
S	**Long run** 0.5 mile Z1 10.0 miles Z2 0.5 mile Z1	Sports drink or gels + water	At least 0.6 g CHO, 0.15 g PRO per kg body weight	

		LEVEL 3 / WEEK 6 / RECOVERY WEEK		
	WORKOUT	NUTRITION DURING WORKOUT	RECOVERY NUTRITION (WITHIN 45:00 OF COMPLETING WORKOUT)	GENERAL DIET
M	**Rest**			4–5 g CHO per kg body weight
T	**Hill repetitions run** 5:00 Z1 10:00 Z2 12 × (0:30 Z5/2:30 Z1) 5:00 Z1	Water, water + electrolytes, or nothing	At least 0.8 g CHO, 0.2 g PRO per kg body weight	
W	**Recovery run** 45:00 Z1	Water, water + electrolytes, or nothing	At least 0.4 g CHO, 0.1 g PRO per kg body weight	
T	**Foundation run** 5:00 Z1 40:00 Z2 5:00 Z1	Water, water + electrolytes, or nothing	At least 0.4 g CHO, 0.1 g PRO per kg body weight	

LEVEL 3 / WEEK 6 / CONTINUED

	WORKOUT	NUTRITION DURING WORKOUT	RECOVERY NUTRITION (WITHIN 45:00 OF COMPLETING WORKOUT)	GENERAL DIET
F	**Fast-finish run** 5:00 Z1 35:00 Z2 10:00 Z3	Water, water + electrolytes, or nothing	At least 0.6 g CHO, 0.15 g PRO per kg body weight	4–5 g CHO per kg body weight
S	**Foundation run** 5:00 Z1 40:00 Z2 5:00 Z1	Water, water + electrolytes, or nothing	At least 0.4 g CHO, 0.1 g PRO per kg body weight	
S	**Long run** 0.5 mile Z1 9.0 miles Z2 0.5 mile Z1	Sports drink or gels + water	At least 0.6 g CHO, 0.15 g PRO per kg body weight	

LEVEL 3 / WEEK 7

	WORKOUT	NUTRITION DURING WORKOUT	RECOVERY NUTRITION (WITHIN 45:00 OF COMPLETING WORKOUT)	GENERAL DIET
M	**Foundation run** 5:00 Z1 40:00 Z2 5:00 Z1 OR Cross-training	Water, water + electrolytes, or nothing	At least 0.4 g CHO, 0.1 g PRO per kg body weight	5–6 g CHO per kg body weight
T	**Hill repetitions run** 5:00 Z1 10:00 Z2 10 × (1:00 Z5/2:30 Z1) 5:00 Z1	Water, water + electrolytes, or nothing	At least 0.8 g CHO, 0.2 g PRO per kg body weight	
W	**Recovery run** 45:00 Z1	Water, water + electrolytes, or nothing	At least 0.4 g CHO, 0.1 g PRO per kg body weight	
T	**Foundation run** 5:00 Z1 40:00 Z2 5:00 Z1	Water, water + electrolytes, or nothing	At least 0.6 g CHO, 0.15 g PRO per kg body weight	
F	**Fast-finish run** 5:00 Z1 35:00 Z2 10:00 Z3	Water, water + electrolytes, or nothing	At least 0.6 g CHO, 0.15 g PRO per kg body weight	
S	**Foundation run** 5:00 Z1 40:00 Z2 5:00 Z1	Water, water + electrolytes, or nothing	At least 0.6 g CHO, 0.12 g PRO per kg body weight	
S	**Long run** 0.5 mile Z1 12.0 miles Z2 0.5 mile Z1	Sports drink or gels + water	At least 0.8 g CHO, 0.2 g PRO per kg body weight	

LEVEL 3 / WEEK 8

	WORKOUT	NUTRITION DURING WORKOUT	RECOVERY NUTRITION (WITHIN 45:00 OF COMPLETING WORKOUT)	GENERAL DIET
M	**Foundation run** 5:00 Z1 40:00 Z2 5:00 Z1 OR Cross-training	Water, water + electrolytes, or nothing	At least 0.4 g CHO, 0.1 g PRO per kg body weight	5–6 g CHO per kg body weight
T	**Hill repetitions run** 5:00 Z1 10:00 Z2 8 × (2:00 Z4/2:30 Z1) 5:00 Z1	Water, water + electrolytes, or nothing	At least 0.8 g CHO, 0.2 g PRO per kg body weight	
W	**Recovery run** 45:00 Z1	Water, water + electrolytes, or nothing	At least 0.4 g CHO, 0.1 g PRO per kg body weight	
T	**Foundation run** 5:00 Z1 40:00 Z2 5:00 Z1	Water, water + electrolytes, or nothing	At least 0.4 g CHO, 0.1 g PRO per kg body weight	
F	**Fast-finish run** 5:00 Z1 40:00 Z2 10:00 Z3	Water, water + electrolytes, or nothing	At least 0.6 g CHO, 0.15 g PRO per kg body weight	
S	**Foundation run** 5:00 Z1 40:00 Z2 5:00 Z1	Water, water + electrolytes, or nothing	At least 0.4 g CHO, 0.1 g PRO per kg body weight	
S	**Long run** 0.5 mile Z1 13.0 miles Z2 0.5 mile Z1	Water, water + electrolytes, or nothing	At least 0.8 g CHO, 0.2 g PRO per kg body weight	

LEVEL 3 / WEEK 9

	WORKOUT	NUTRITION DURING WORKOUT	RECOVERY NUTRITION (WITHIN 45:00 OF COMPLETING WORKOUT)	GENERAL DIET
M	**Rest**			Day 1 of 3-day fat-loading test (optional)
T	**Interval run** 5:00 Z1 10:00 Z2 7 × (2:00 Z4/2:30 Z1) 5:00 Z1	Water, water + electrolytes, or nothing	At least 0.8 g CHO, 0.2 g PRO per kg body weight	Day 2 of 3-day fat-loading test (optional)
W	**Recovery run** 45:00 Z1	Water, water + electrolytes, or nothing	At least 0.4 g CHO, 0.1 g PRO per kg body weight	Day 3 of 3-day fat-loading test (optional)

	LEVEL 3 / WEEK 9 / CONTINUED			
	WORKOUT	NUTRITION DURING WORKOUT	RECOVERY NUTRITION (WITHIN 45:00 OF COMPLETING WORKOUT)	GENERAL DIET
T	**Foundation run** 5:00 Z1 40:00 Z2 5:00 Z1	Water, water + electrolytes, or nothing	At least 0.6 g CHO, 0.15 g PRO per kg body weight	5–6 g CHO per kg body weight
F	**Fast-finish run** 5:00 Z1 40:00 Z2 10:00 Z3	Water, water + electrolytes, or nothing	At least 0.6 g CHO, 0.15 g PRO per kg body weight	
S	**Recovery run** 50:00 Z1	Water, water + electrolytes, or nothing	At least 0.6 g CHO, 0.15 g PRO per kg body weight	
S	**Long run** 0.5 mile Z1 10.0 miles Z2 0.5 mile Z1	Sports drink or gels + water	At least 0.6 g CHO, 0.15 g PRO per kg body weight	

	LEVEL 3 / WEEK 10			
	WORKOUT	NUTRITION DURING WORKOUT	RECOVERY NUTRITION (WITHIN 45:00 OF COMPLETING WORKOUT)	GENERAL DIET
M	**Foundation run** 5:00 Z1 45:00 Z2 5:00 Z1 OR Cross-training	Water, water + electrolytes, or nothing	At least 0.6 g CHO, 0.15 g PRO per kg body weight	5–6 g CHO per kg body weight
T	**Interval run** 5:00 Z1 10:00 Z2 9 × (2:00 Z4/2:30 Z1) 5:00 Z1	Water, water + electrolytes, or nothing	At least 0.8 g CHO, 0.2 g PRO per kg body weight	
W	**Recovery run** 50:00 Z1	Water, water + electrolytes, or nothing	At least 0.4 g CHO, 0.1 g PRO per kg body weight	
T	**Foundation run** 5:00 Z1 45:00 Z2 5:00 Z1	Water, water + electrolytes, or nothing	At least 0.6 g CHO, 0.15 g PRO per kg body weight	
F	**Fast-finish run** 5:00 Z1 40:00 Z2 15:00 Z3	Water, water + electrolytes, or nothing	At least 0.8 g CHO, 0.20 g PRO per kg body weight	
S	**Foundation run** 5:00 Z1 45:00 Z2 5:00 Z1	Water, water + electrolytes, or nothing	At least 0.6 g CHO, 0.15 g PRO per kg body weight	
S	**Long run** 0.5 mile Z1 14.0 miles Z2 0.5 mile Z1	Water, water + electrolytes, or nothing	At least 0.8 g CHO, 0.2 g PRO per kg body weight	

LEVEL 3 / WEEK 11			
WORKOUT	**NUTRITION DURING WORKOUT**	**RECOVERY NUTRITION (WITHIN 45:00 OF COMPLETING WORKOUT)**	**GENERAL DIET**
M Foundation run 5:00 Z1 45:00 Z2 5:00 Z1 OR Cross-training	Water, water + electrolytes, or nothing	At least 0.6 g CHO, 0.15 g PRO per kg body weight	5–6 g CHO per kg body weight
T Interval run 5:00 Z1 10:00 Z2 6 × (3:00 Z4/2:30 Z1) 5:00 Z1	Water, water + electrolytes, or nothing	At least 0.8 g CHO, 0.2 g PRO per kg body weight	
W Recovery run 50:00 Z1	Water, water + electrolytes, or nothing	At least 0.4 g CHO, 0.1 g PRO per kg body weight	
T Foundation run 5:00 Z1 45:00 Z2 5:00 Z1	Water, water + electrolytes, or nothing	At least 0.6 g CHO, 0.15 g PRO per kg body weight	
F Tempo run 5:00 Z1 10:00 Z2 30:00 Z3 10:00 Z2 5:00 Z1	Water, water + electrolytes, or nothing	At least 0.8 g CHO, 0.2 g PRO per kg body weight	
S Recovery run 50:00 Z1	Water, water + electrolytes, or nothing	At least 0.4 g CHO, 0.1 g PRO per kg body weight	
S Long run 0.5 mile Z1 13.0 miles Z2 0.5 mile Z1	Sports drink or gels + water	At least 0.8 g CHO, 0.2 g PRO per kg body weight	

LEVEL 3 / WEEK 12 / RECOVERY WEEK			
WORKOUT	**NUTRITION DURING WORKOUT**	**RECOVERY NUTRITION (WITHIN 45:00 OF COMPLETING WORKOUT)**	**GENERAL DIET**
M Rest			5–6 g CHO per kg body weight
T Hill repetitions run 5:00 Z1 10:00 Z2 10 × (0:30 Z5/2:30 Z1) 5:00 Z1	Water, water + electrolytes, or nothing	At least 0.6 g CHO, 0.15 g PRO per kg body weight	
W Recovery run 50:00 Z1	Water, water + electrolytes, or nothing	At least 0.4 g CHO, 0.1 g PRO per kg body weight	
T Foundation run 5:00 Z1 35:00 Z2 5:00 Z1	Water, water + electrolytes, or nothing	At least 0.4 g CHO, 0.1 g PRO per kg body weight	

	LEVEL 3 / WEEK 12 / RECOVERY WEEK / CONTINUED			
	WORKOUT	**NUTRITION DURING WORKOUT**	**RECOVERY NUTRITION (WITHIN 45:00 OF COMPLETING WORKOUT)**	**GENERAL DIET**
F	**Tempo run** 5:00 Z1 10:00 Z2 20:00 Z3 10:00 Z2 5:00 Z1	Water, water + electrolytes, or nothing	At least 0.8 g CHO, 0.2 g PRO per kg body weight	5–6 g CHO per kg body weight
S	**Foundation run** 5:00 Z1 35:00 Z2 5:00 Z1	Water, water + electrolytes, or nothing	At least 0.4 g CHO, 0.1 g PRO per kg body weight	
S	**Long run with fast finish** 0.5 mile Z1 9.5 miles Z2 1.0 mile Z3	Water, water + electrolytes, or nothing	At least 0.8 g CHO, 0.2 g PRO per kg body weight	

	LEVEL 3 / WEEK 13			
	WORKOUT	**NUTRITION DURING WORKOUT**	**RECOVERY NUTRITION (WITHIN 45:00 OF COMPLETING WORKOUT)**	**GENERAL DIET**
M	**Foundation run** 5:00 Z1 50:00 Z2 5:00 Z1 OR Cross-training	Water, water + electrolytes, or nothing	At least 0.8 g CHO, 0.2 g PRO per kg body weight	5–6 g CHO per kg body weight
T	**Interval run** 5:00 Z1 10:00 Z2 5 × (4:00 Z4/2:30 Z1) 5:00 Z1	Water, water + electrolytes, or nothing	At least 0.8 g CHO, 0.2 g PRO per kg body weight	
W	**Recovery run** 60:00 Z1	Water, water + electrolytes, or nothing	At least 0.6 g CHO, 0.15 g PRO per kg body weight	
T	**Foundation run** 5:00 Z1 50:00 Z2 5:00 Z1	Water, water + electrolytes, or nothing	At least 0.6 g CHO, 0.15 g PRO per kg body weight	
F	**Tempo run** 5:00 Z1 10:00 Z2 35:00 Z3 10:00 Z2 5:00 Z1	Water, water + electrolytes, or nothing	At least 0.8 g CHO, 0.2 g PRO per kg body weight	
S	**Recovery run** 60:00 Z1	Water, water + electrolytes, or nothing	At least 0.6 g CHO, 0.15 g PRO per kg body weight	
S	**Long run with fast finish** 0.5 mile Z1 13.5 miles Z2 1.0 mile Z3	Water, water + electrolytes, or nothing	At least 1.0 g CHO, 0.25 g PRO per kg body weight	

		LEVEL 3 / WEEK 14		
	WORKOUT	NUTRITION DURING WORKOUT	RECOVERY NUTRITION (WITHIN 45:00 OF COMPLETING WORKOUT)	GENERAL DIET
M	**Recovery run** 60:00 Z1	Water, water + electrolytes, or nothing	At least 0.6 g CHO, 0.15 g PRO per kg body weight	5–6 g CHO per kg body weight
T	**Speed-play run** 5:00 Z1 5:00 Z2 1:30 Z2 2:30 Z1 3:00 Z4 2:00 Z1 5:00 Z3 2:00 Z1 3:00 Z4 2:00 Z1 1:30 Z5 2:30 Z1 5:00 Z2 5:00 Z1	Water, water + electrolytes, or nothing	At least 0.8 g CHO, 0.2 g PRO per kg body weight	
W	**Recovery run** 60:00 Z1	Water, water + electrolytes, or nothing	At least 0.4 g CHO, 0.1 g PRO per kg body weight	
T	**Foundation run** 5:00 Z1 35:00 Z2 5:00 Z1	Water, water + electrolytes, or nothing	At least 0.4 g CHO, 0.1 g PRO per kg body weight	
F	**Tempo run** 5:00 Z1 5:00 Z2 40:00 Z3 5:00 Z2 5:00 Z1	Water, water + electrolytes, or nothing	At least 0.8 g CHO, 0.2 g PRO per kg body weight	
S	**Recovery run** 60:00 Z1	Water, water + electrolytes, or nothing	At least 0.6 g CHO, 0.15 g PRO per kg body weight	
S	**Simulator** 0.5 mile Z1 1.5 mile Z2 13.1 km (8.1 miles) @ half-marathon race pace 1.0 mile Z1	Practice race nutrition plan	At least 0.8 g CHO, 0.2 g PRO per kg body weight	

	WORKOUT	NUTRITION DURING WORKOUT	RECOVERY NUTRITION (WITHIN 45:00 OF COMPLETING WORKOUT)	GENERAL DIET
	LEVEL 3 / WEEK 15 / TAPER PERIOD			
M	Rest			Reduce caloric intake by amount equal to average per-day reduction in calories burned through training in taper period compared to Week 14 Start 10-day fat-loading period (65 percent of calories from fat) (optional)
T	Interval run 5:00 Z1 5:00 Z2 2 × (1:00 Z5/ 2:00 Z1) 2:00 Z4 2:00 Z1 5:00 Z3 2:00 Z1 2:00 Z4 2:00 Z1 2 × (1:00 Z5/ 2:00 Z1) 5:00 Z2 5:00 Z1	Water, water + electrolytes, or nothing	At least 0.6 g CHO, 0.15 g PRO per kg body weight	Day 2 of reduced calorie intake Day 2 of 10-day fat-loading period (65 percent of calories from fat) (optional)
W	Recovery run 45:00 Z1	Water, water + electrolytes, or nothing	At least 0.4 g CHO, 0.1 g PRO per kg body weight	Day 3 of reduced calorie intake Day 3 of 10-day fat-loading period (65 percent of calories from fat) (optional)
T	Foundation run 5:00 Z1 35:00 Z2 5:00 Z1	Water, water + electrolytes, or nothing	At least 0.4 g CHO, 0.1 g PRO per kg body weight	Day 4 of reduced calorie intake Day 4 of 10-day fat-loading period (65 percent of calories from fat) (optional)
F	Tempo run 5:00 Z1 10:00 Z2 30:00 Z3 10:00 Z2 5:00 Z1	Water, water + electrolytes, or nothing	At least 0.8 g CHO, 0.2 g PRO per kg body weight	Day 5 of reduced calorie intake Day 5 of 10-day fat-loading period (65 percent of calories from fat) (optional)
S	Recovery run 45:00 Z1	Water, water + electrolytes, or nothing	At least 0.4 g CHO, 0.1 g PRO per kg body weight	Day 6 of reduced calorie intake Day 6 of 10-day fat-loading period (65 percent of calories from fat) (optional)
S	Long run with fast finish 0.5 mile Z1 11.5 miles Z2 1.0 mile Z3	Sports drink or gels + water	At least 0.8 g CHO, 0.2 g PRO per kg body weight	Day 7 of reduced calorie intake Start 7-day caffeine fast (optional) Day 7 of 10-day fat-loading period (65 percent of calories from fat) (optional)

	WORKOUT	NUTRITION DURING WORKOUT	RECOVERY NUTRITION (WITHIN 45:00 OF COMPLETING WORKOUT)	GENERAL DIET
M	**Recovery run** 45:00 Z1	Water, water + electrolytes, or nothing	At least 0.4 g CHO, 0.1 g PRO per kg	Day 8 of reduced calorie intake Day 8 of 10-day fat-loading period (65 percent of calories from fat) (optional) OR Start 5-day fat-loading period (optional) Day 2 of 7-day caffeine fast (optional)
T	**Speed-play run** 5:00 Z1 10:00 Z2 8 × (0:30 Z4/ 2:30 Z2) 5:00 Z1	Water, water + electrolytes, or nothing	At least 0.4 g CHO, 0.1 g PRO per kg body weight	Day 9 of reduced calorie intake Day 9 of 10-day fat-loading period (65 percent of calories from fat) (optional) OR Day 2 of 5-day fat-loading period (optional) Day 3 of 7-day caffeine fast (optional)
W	**Recovery run** 45:00 Z1	Water, water + electrolytes, or nothing	At least 0.4 g CHO, 0.1 g PRO per kg body weight	Day 10 of reduced calorie intake Day 10 of 10-day fat-loading period (65 percent of calories from fat) (optional) OR Day 3 of 5-day fat-loading period (optional) Day 4 of 7-day caffeine fast (optional)
T	**Fast finish run** 5:00 Z1 20:00 Z2 10:00 Z3	Water, water + electrolytes, or nothing	At least 0.4 g CHO, 0.1 g PRO per kg body weight	Day 11 of reduced calorie intake Day 1 of 3-day carbo-loading period (70 percent of calories from CHO) OR Day 4 of 5-day fat-loading period (optional) Day 5 of 7-day caffeine fast (optional)

LEVEL 3 / WEEK 16 / TAPER PERIOD

			LEVEL 3 / WEEK 16 / TAPER PERIOD / CONTINUED	
	WORKOUT	**NUTRITION DURING WORKOUT**	**RECOVERY NUTRITION (WITHIN 45:00 OF COMPLETING WORKOUT)**	**GENERAL DIET**
F	**Recovery run** 30:00 Z1	Water, water + electrolytes, or nothing	At least 0.4 g CHO, 0.1 g PRO per kg	Day 12 of reduced calorie intake Day 2 of 3-day carbo-loading period (70 percent of calories from CHO) OR Day 5 of 5-day fat-loading period (optional) Day 6 of 7-day caffeine fast (optional)
S	**Speed-play run** 5:00 Z1 5:00 Z2 4 × (0:30 Z4/ 1:30 Z2) 5:00 Z1	Water, water + electrolytes, or nothing	At least 0.4 g CHO, 0.1 g PRO per kg	Day 3 of 3-day carbo-loading period (70 percent of calories from CHO) OR Day 1 of 1-day carbo-loading period (10 g CHO per kg body weight) (optional) Day 7 of 7-day caffeine fast (optional)
S	**Half marathon**	Race nutrition plan	Anything you want!	Prerace nutrition plan

NUTRITION-TRAINING PLANS FOR THE MARATHON

Twenty weeks is an appropriate amount of time to train for a marathon, assuming you're not already close to peak fitness. If you're a first-timer, twenty weeks is just enough time to develop the basic endurance you'll need to go the distance. If you're an experienced runner aiming for a new personal best, twenty weeks is long enough to take your running to a whole new level yet not so long that you're likely to burn out.

Each of the three integrated training and nutrition plans for the marathon presented in this chapter is twenty weeks in length. The Level 1 plan is for first-timers, the Level 2 plan is for more experienced runners seeking improvement, and the Level 3 plan is for advanced competitive runners. All of the general information I shared in the introduction to the half-marathon plans in the preceding chapter applies to these plans as well, so be sure to read that (pages 191–192).

If you'd like more personalized coaching, interactive audio versions of the plans are available at pearsports.com. To use them you will need to own a PEAR Sports device such as the Square One. Simply download the workouts onto the device—which includes a heart-rate

229

monitor, a foot pod for speed and distance tracking, a mini computer, and headphones—and follow my verbal instructions as I guide you through each workout and give you tips on diet, injury prevention, motivation, and more.

LEVEL 1 MARATHON PLAN

This twenty-week integrated training and nutrition plan for the marathon is a good fit for runners who are training for their first marathon or who need or prefer a lower-volume approach to training for whatever reason. The schedule prescribes four runs per week plus two optional cross-training workouts. You should be able to comfortably run 4 miles before you start the program.

The hardest week of training is Week 18, which includes a marathon Simulator (26.2 km at marathon race pace) and a total of approximately five hours of running. Weeks 4, 8, 12, and 16 are reduced-volume recovery weeks. The program ends with a one-week taper.

TABLE 11.1 *LEVEL 1 MARATHON PLAN*

LEVEL 1 / WEEK 1

	WORKOUT	NUTRITION DURING WORKOUT	RECOVERY NUTRITION (WITHIN 45:00 OF COMPLETING WORKOUT)	GENERAL DIET
M	Rest			3–4 g CHO per kg body weight
T	**Foundation run** 5:00 Z1 15:00 Z2 5:00 Z1	Water, water + electrolytes, or nothing	At least 0.4 g CHO, 0.1 g PRO per kg body weight	
W	**Cross-training** Optional			
T	**Foundation run** 5:00 Z1 15:00 Z2 5:00 Z1	Water, water + electrolytes, or nothing	At least 0.4 g CHO, 0.1 g PRO per kg body weight	
F	**Foundation run** 5:00 Z1 15:00 Z2 5:00 Z1	Water, water + electrolytes, or nothing	At least 0.4 g CHO, 0.1 g PRO per kg body weight	
S	**Cross-training** Optional			
S	**Long run** 0.5 mile Z1 3.0 miles Z2 0.5 mile Z1	Water, water + electrolytes, or nothing	At least 0.4 g CHO, 0.1 g PRO per kg body weight	

LEVEL 1 / WEEK 2

	WORKOUT	NUTRITION DURING WORKOUT	RECOVERY NUTRITION (WITHIN 45:00 OF COMPLETING WORKOUT)	GENERAL DIET
M	Rest			3–4 g CHO per kg body weight
T	**Foundation run** 5:00 Z1 20:00 Z2 5:00 Z1	Water, water + electrolytes, or nothing	At least 0.4 g CHO, 0.1 g PRO per kg body weight	
W	**Cross-training** Optional			
T	**Foundation run** 5:00 Z1 20:00 Z2 5:00 Z1	Water, water + electrolytes, or nothing	At least 0.4 g CHO, 0.1 g PRO per kg body weight	
F	**Foundation run** 5:00 Z1 20:00 Z2 5:00 Z1	Water, water + electrolytes, or nothing	At least 0.4 g CHO, 0.1 g PRO per kg body weight	
S	**Cross-training** Optional			
S	**Long run** 0.5 mile Z1 4.0 miles Z2 0.5 mile Z1	Water, water + electrolytes, or nothing	At least 0.4 g CHO, 0.1 g PRO per kg body weight	

	LEVEL 1 / WEEK 3			
	WORKOUT	**NUTRITION DURING WORKOUT**	**RECOVERY NUTRITION (WITHIN 45:00 OF COMPLETING WORKOUT)**	**GENERAL DIET**
M	**Rest**			3–4 g CHO per kg body weight
T	**Speed-play run** 5:00 Z1 5:00 Z2 6 × (0:15 Z5/ 2:45 Z2) 5:00 Z1	Water, water + electrolytes, or nothing	At least 0.4 g CHO, 0.1 g PRO per kg body weight	
W	**Cross-training** Optional			
T	**Foundation run** 5:00 Z1 20:00 Z2 5:00 Z1	Water, water + electrolytes, or nothing	At least 0.4 g CHO, 0.1 g PRO per kg body weight	
F	**Fast-finish run** 5:00 Z1 20:00 Z2 5:00 Z3	Water, water + electrolytes, or nothing	At least 0.4 g CHO, 0.1 g PRO per kg body weight	
S	**Cross-training** Optional			
S	**Long run** 0.5 mile Z1 5.0 miles Z2 0.5 mile Z1	Water, water + electrolytes, or nothing	At least 0.4 g CHO, 0.1 g PRO per kg body weight	

	LEVEL 1 / WEEK 4 / RECOVERY WEEK			
	WORKOUT	**NUTRITION DURING WORKOUT**	**RECOVERY NUTRITION (WITHIN 45:00 OF COMPLETING WORKOUT)**	**GENERAL DIET**
M	**Rest**			3–4 g CHO per kg body weight
T	**Speed-play run** 5:00 Z1 5:00 Z2 5 × (0:15 5/2:45 Z2) 5:00 Z1	Water, water + electrolytes, or nothing	At least 0.4 g CHO, 0.1 g PRO per kg body weight	
W	**Cross-training** Optional			
T	**Foundation run** 5:00 Z1 20:00 Z2 5:00 Z1	Water, water + electrolytes, or nothing	At least 0.4 g CHO, 0.1 g PRO per kg body weight	
F	**Fast-finish run** 5:00 Z1 20:00 Z2 5:00 Z3	Water, water + electrolytes, or nothing	At least 0.4 g CHO, 0.1 g PRO per kg body weight	
S	**Cross-training** Optional			
S	**Long run** 0.5 mile Z1 4.0 miles Z2 0.5 mile Z1	Water, water + electrolytes, or nothing	At least 0.4 g CHO, 0.1 g PRO per kg body weight	

LEVEL 1 / WEEK 5				
	WORKOUT	**NUTRITION DURING WORKOUT**	**RECOVERY NUTRITION (WITHIN 45:00 OF COMPLETING WORKOUT)**	**GENERAL DIET**
M	Rest			3–4 g CHO per kg body weight
T	**Hill repetitions run** 5:00 Z1 5:00 Z2 8 × (0:30 Z5/2:30 Z1) 5:00 Z1	Water, water + electrolytes, or nothing	At least 0.4 g CHO, 0.1 g PRO per kg body weight	
W	**Cross-training** Optional			
T	**Foundation run** 5:00 Z1 30:00 Z2 5:00 Z1	Water, water + electrolytes, or nothing	At least 0.4 g CHO, 0.1 g PRO per kg body weight	
F	**Fast-finish run** 5:00 Z1 30:00 Z2 5:00 Z3	Water, water + electrolytes, or nothing	At least 0.4 g CHO, 0.1 g PRO per kg body weight	
S	**Cross-training** Optional			
S	**Long run** 0.5 mile Z1 6.0 miles Z2 0.5 mile Z1	Sports drink or gels + water	At least 0.4 g CHO, 0.1 g PRO per kg body weight	

LEVEL 1 / WEEK 6				
	WORKOUT	**NUTRITION DURING WORKOUT**	**RECOVERY NUTRITION (WITHIN 45:00 OF COMPLETING WORKOUT)**	**GENERAL DIET**
M	Rest			3–4 g CHO per kg body weight
T	**Hill repetitions run** 5:00 Z1 5:00 Z2 7 × (0:30 Z5/2:30 Z1) 5:00 Z1	Water, water + electrolytes, or nothing	At least 0.6 g CHO, 0.1 g PRO per kg body weight	
W	**Cross-training** Optional			
T	**Foundation run** 5:00 Z1 25:00 Z2 5:00 Z1	Water, water + electrolytes, or nothing	At least 0.4 g CHO, 0.1 g PRO per kg body weight	
F	**Fast-finish run** 5:00 Z1 20:00 Z2 10:00 Z3	Water, water + electrolytes, or nothing	At least 0.4 g CHO, 0.1 g PRO per kg body weight	
S	**Cross-training** Optional			
S	**Long run** 0.5 mile Z1 7.0 miles Z2 0.5 mile Z1	Water or water + electrolytes	At least 0.6 g CHO, 0.15 g PRO per kg body weight	

LEVEL 1 / WEEK 7

	WORKOUT	NUTRITION DURING WORKOUT	RECOVERY NUTRITION (WITHIN 45:00 OF COMPLETING WORKOUT)	GENERAL DIET
M	Rest			3–4 g CHO per kg body weight
T	**Hill repetitions run** 5:00 Z1 5:00 Z2 8 × (1:00 Z5/2:30 Z1) 5:00 Z1	Water, water + electrolytes, or nothing	At least 0.6 g CHO, 0.1 g PRO per kg body weight	
W	**Cross-training** Optional			
T	**Foundation run** 5:00 Z1 30:00 Z2 5:00 Z1	Water, water + electrolytes, or nothing	At least 0.4 g CHO, 0.1 g PRO per kg body weight	
F	**Fast-finish run** 5:00 Z1 25:00 Z2 10:00 Z3	Water, water + electrolytes, or nothing	At least 0.4 g CHO, 0.1 g PRO per kg body weight	
S	**Cross-training** Optional			
S	**Long run** 0.5 mile Z1 8.0 miles Z2 0.5 mile Z1	Sports drink or gels + water	At least 0.6 g CHO, 0.15 g PRO per kg body weight	

LEVEL 1 / WEEK 8 / RECOVERY WEEK

	WORKOUT	NUTRITION DURING WORKOUT	RECOVERY NUTRITION (WITHIN 45:00 OF COMPLETING WORKOUT)	GENERAL DIET
M	Rest			3–4 g CHO per kg body weight
T	**Hill repetitions run** 5:00 Z1 5:00 Z2 8 × (0:30 Z5/2:30 Z1) 5:00 Z1	Water, water + electrolytes, or nothing	At least 0.6 g CHO, 0.15 g PRO per kg body weight	
W	**Cross-training** Optional			
T	**Foundation run** 5:00 Z1 30:00 Z2 5:00 Z1	Water, water + electrolytes, or nothing	At least 0.4 g CHO, 0.1 g PRO per kg body weight	
F	**Fast-finish run** 5:00 Z1 30:00 Z2 5:00 Z3	Water, water + electrolytes, or nothing	At least 0.4 g CHO, 0.1 g PRO per kg body weight	
S	**Cross-training** Optional			
S	**Long run** 0.5 mile Z1 7.0 miles Z2 0.5 mile Z1	Water or water + electrolytes	At least 0.6 g CHO, 0.15 g PRO per kg body weight	

LEVEL 1 / WEEK 9

	WORKOUT	NUTRITION DURING WORKOUT	RECOVERY NUTRITION (WITHIN 45:00 OF COMPLETING WORKOUT)	GENERAL DIET
M	Rest			3–4 g CHO per kg body weight
T	Interval run 5:00 Z1 5:00 Z2 8 × (1:00 Z5/2:00 Z1) 5:00 Z1	Water, water + electrolytes, or nothing	At least 0.6 g CHO, 0.15 g PRO per kg body weight	
W	Cross-training Optional			
T	Foundation run 5:00 Z1 35:00 Z2 5:00 Z1	Water, water + electrolytes, or nothing	At least 0.4 g CHO, 0.1 g PRO per kg body weight	
F	Fast-finish run 5:00 Z1 30:00 Z2 10:00 Z3	Water, water + electrolytes, or nothing	At least 0.6 g CHO, 0.15 g PRO per kg body weight	
S	Cross-training Optional			
S	Long run 0.5 mile Z1 9.0 miles Z2 0.5 mile Z1	Water or water + electrolytes	At least 0.6 g CHO, 0.15 g PRO per kg body weight	

LEVEL 1 / WEEK 10

	WORKOUT	NUTRITION DURING WORKOUT	RECOVERY NUTRITION (WITHIN 45:00 OF COMPLETING WORKOUT)	GENERAL DIET
M	Rest			3–4 g CHO per kg body weight
T	Interval run 5:00 Z1 5:00 Z2 10 × (1:00 Z5/2:00 Z1) 5:00 Z1	Water, water + electrolytes, or nothing	At least 0.6 g CHO, 0.15 g PRO per kg body weight	
W	Cross-training Optional			
T	Foundation run 5:00 Z1 35:00 Z2 5:00 Z1	Water, water + electrolytes, or nothing	At least 0.4 g CHO, 0.1 g PRO per kg body weight	
F	Fast-finish run 5:00 Z1 30:00 Z2 10:00 Z3	Water, water + electrolytes, or nothing	At least 0.6 g CHO, 0.15 g PRO per kg body weight	
S	Cross-training Optional			
S	Long run 0.5 mile Z1 10.0 miles Z2 0.5 mile Z1	Sports drink or gels + water	At least 0.6 g CHO, 0.15 g PRO per kg body weight	

			LEVEL 1 / WEEK 11	
	WORKOUT	NUTRITION DURING WORKOUT	RECOVERY NUTRITION (WITHIN 45:00 OF COMPLETING WORKOUT)	GENERAL DIET
M	Rest			3–4 g CHO per kg body weight
T	Interval run 5:00 Z1 5:00 Z2 8 × (1:30 Z5/2:30 Z1) 5:00 Z1	Water, water + electrolytes, or nothing	At least 0.6 g CHO, 0.15 g PRO per kg body weight	
W	Cross-training Optional			
T	Foundation run 5:00 Z1 35:00 Z2 5:00 Z1	Water, water + electrolytes, or nothing	At least 0.4 g CHO, 0.1 g PRO per kg body weight	
F	Fast-finish run 5:00 Z1 28:00 Z2 12:00 Z3	Water, water + electrolytes, or nothing	At least 0.6 g CHO, 0.15 g PRO per kg body weight	
S	Cross-training Optional			
S	Long run 0.5 mile Z1 11.0 miles Z2 0.5 mile	If anticipated run duration is less than 2 hours: water or water + electrolytes If anticipated run duration is more than 2 hours: sports drink or gels + water	At least 0.8 g CHO, 0.2 g PRO per kg body weight	

			LEVEL 1 / WEEK 12 / RECOVERY WEEK	
	WORKOUT	NUTRITION DURING WORKOUT	RECOVERY NUTRITION (WITHIN 45:00 OF COMPLETING WORKOUT)	GENERAL DIET
M	Rest			Day 1 of 3-day fat-loading test (optional)
T	Hill repetitions run 5:00 Z1 5:00 Z2 5 × (1:00 Z5/ 2:30 Z1) 5:00 Z1	Water, water + electrolytes, or nothing	At least 0.4 g CHO, 0.1 g PRO per kg body weight	Day 2 of 3-day fat-loading test (optional)
W	Cross-training Optional			Day 3 of 3-day fat-loading test (optional)
T	Foundation run 5:00 Z1 30:00 Z2 5:00 Z1	Water, water + electrolytes, or nothing	At least 0.4 g CHO, 0.1 g PRO per kg body weight	3–4 g CHO per kg body weight

LEVEL 1 / WEEK 12 / RECOVERY WEEK / CONTINUED

	WORKOUT	NUTRITION DURING WORKOUT	RECOVERY NUTRITION (WITHIN 45:00 OF COMPLETING WORKOUT)	GENERAL DIET
F	**Fast-finish run** 5:00 Z1 30:00 Z2 5:00 Z3	Water, water + electrolytes, or nothing	At least 0.4 g CHO, 0.1 g PRO per kg body weight	3–4 g CHO per kg body weight
S	**Cross-training** Optional			
S	**Long run** 0.5 mile Z1 9.0 miles Z2 0.5 mile Z1	Water, water + electrolytes, or nothing	At least 0.6 g CHO, 0.15 g PRO per kg body weight	

LEVEL 1 / WEEK 13

	WORKOUT	NUTRITION DURING WORKOUT	RECOVERY NUTRITION (WITHIN 45:00 OF COMPLETING WORKOUT)	GENERAL DIET
M	**Rest**			3–4 g CHO per kg body weight
T	**Speed-play run** 5:00 Z1 5:00 Z2 6 × (2:00 Z4/2:30 Z1) 5:00 Z1	Water, water + electrolytes, or nothing	At least 0.8 g CHO, 0.2 g PRO per kg body weight	
W	**Cross-training** Optional			
T	**Foundation run** 5:00 Z1 35:00 Z2 5:00 Z1	Water, water + electrolytes, or nothing	At least 0.4 g CHO, 0.1 g PRO per kg body weight	
F	**Tempo run** 5:00 Z1 10:00 Z2 14:00 Z3 10:00 Z2 5:00 Z1	Water, water + electrolytes, or nothing	At least 0.6 g CHO, 0.15 g PRO per kg body weight	
S	**Cross-training** Optional			
S	**Long run** 0.5 mile Z1 13.0 miles Z2 0.5 mile Z1	If anticipated run duration is less than 2 hours: water or water + electrolytes If anticipated run duration is more than 2 hours: sports drink or gels + water	At least 0.8 g CHO, 0.2 g PRO per kg body weight	

LEVEL 1 / WEEK 14				
	WORKOUT	NUTRITION DURING WORKOUT	RECOVERY NUTRITION (WITHIN 45:00 OF COMPLETING WORKOUT)	GENERAL DIET
M	Rest			3–4 g CHO per kg body weight
T	**Speed-play run** 5:00 Z1 7:30 Z2 5 × (3:00 Z4/2:30 Z1) 5:00 Z1	Water, water + electrolytes, or nothing	At least 0.6 g CHO, 0.15 g PRO per kg body weight	
W	**Cross-training** Optional			
T	**Foundation run** 5:00 Z1 35:00 Z2 5:00 Z1	Water, water + electrolytes, or nothing	At least 0.4 g CHO, 0.1 g PRO per kg body weight	
F	**Tempo run** 5:00 Z1 10:00 Z2 16:00 Z3 10:00 Z2 5:00 Z1	Water, water + electrolytes, or nothing	At least 0.6 g CHO, 0.15 g PRO per kg body weight	
S	**Cross-training** Optional			
S	**Long run** 0.5 mile Z1 15.0 miles Z2 0.5 mile Z1	If anticipated run duration is less than 2 hours: water or water + electrolytes If anticipated run duration is more than 2 hours: sports drink or gels + water	At least 1.0 g CHO, 0.2 g PRO per kg body weight	

LEVEL 1 / WEEK 15				
	WORKOUT	NUTRITION DURING WORKOUT	RECOVERY NUTRITION (WITHIN 45:00 OF COMPLETING WORKOUT)	GENERAL DIET
M	Rest			4–5 g CHO per kg body weight
T	**Speed-play run** 5:00 Z1 10:00 Z2 4 × (4:00 Z4/3:00 Z1) 5:00 Z1	Water, water + electrolytes, or nothing	At least 0.6 g CHO, 0.15 g PRO per kg body weight	
W	**Cross-training** Optional			
T	**Foundation run** 5:00 Z1 35:00 Z2 5:00 Z1	Water, water + electrolytes, or nothing	At least 0.4 g CHO, 0.1 g PRO per kg body weight	

LEVEL 1 / WEEK 15 / CONTINUED

	WORKOUT	NUTRITION DURING WORKOUT	RECOVERY NUTRITION (WITHIN 45:00 OF COMPLETING WORKOUT)	GENERAL DIET
F	**Tempo run** 5:00 Z1 10:00 Z2 18:00 Z3 10:00 Z2 5:00 Z1	Water, water + electrolytes, or nothing	At least 0.6 g CHO, 0.15 g PRO per kg body weight	4–5 g CHO per kg body weight
S	**Cross-training** Optional			
S	**Long run** 0.5 mile Z1 17.0 miles Z2 0.5 mile Z1	Sports drink or gels + water	At least 1.0 g CHO, 0.25 g PRO per kg body weight	

LEVEL 1 / WEEK 16 / RECOVERY WEEK

	WORKOUT	NUTRITION DURING WORKOUT	RECOVERY NUTRITION (WITHIN 45:00 OF COMPLETING WORKOUT)	GENERAL DIET
M	**Rest**			3–4 g CHO per kg body weight
T	**Hill repetitions run** 5:00 Z1 10:00 Z2 5 × (2:00 Z4/2.30 Z1) 5:00 Z1	Water, water + electrolytes, or nothing	At least 1.1 g CHO, 0.25 g PRO per kg body weight	
W	**Cross-training** Optional			
T	**Foundation run** 5:00 Z1 35:00 Z2 5:00 Z1	Water, water + electrolytes, or nothing	At least 0.4 g CHO, 0.1 g PRO per kg body weight	
F	**Fast-finish run** 5:00 Z1 25:00 Z2 10:00 Z3	Water, water + electrolytes, or nothing	At least 0.4 g CHO, 0.1 g PRO per kg body weight	
S	**Cross-training** Optional			
S	**Long run** 0.5 mile Z1 12.0 miles Z2 0.5 mile Z1	If anticipated run duration is less than 2 hours: water or water + electrolytes If anticipated run duration is more than 2 hours: sports drink or gels + water	At least 0.6 g CHO, 0.15 g PRO per kg body weight	

	LEVEL 1 / WEEK 17			
	WORKOUT	NUTRITION DURING WORKOUT	RECOVERY NUTRITION (WITHIN 45:00 OF COMPLETING WORKOUT)	GENERAL DIET
M	Rest			4–5 g CHO per kg body weight
T	**Speed-play run** 5:00 Z1 5:00 Z2 1:00 Z5 2:00 Z1 2:00 Z4 2:00 Z1 3:00 Z3 2:00 Z1 2:00 Z4 2:00 Z1 1:00 Z5 2:00 Z1 5:00 Z2 5:00 Z1	Water, water + electrolytes, or nothing	At least 0.6 g CHO, 0.15 g PRO per kg body weight	
W	**Cross-training** Optional			
T	**Foundation run** 5:00 Z1 35:00 Z2 5:00 Z1	Water, water + electrolytes, or nothing	At least 0.4 g CHO, 0.15 g PRO per kg body weight	
F	**Tempo run** 5:00 Z1 5:00 Z2 15:00 Z3 5:00 Z2 5:00 Z1	Water, water + electrolytes, or nothing	At least 0.6 g CHO, 0.15 g PRO per kg body weight	
S	**Cross-training** Optional			
S	**Long run** 0.5 mile Z1 19.0 miles Z2 0.5 mile Z1	Sports drink or gels + water	At least 1.2 g CHO, 0.3 g PRO per kg body weight	

	LEVEL 1 / WEEK 18			
	WORKOUT	NUTRITION DURING WORKOUT	RECOVERY NUTRITION (WITHIN 45:00 OF COMPLETING WORKOUT)	GENERAL DIET
M	Rest			4–5 g CHO per kg body weight
T	**Speed-play run** 5:00 Z1 5:00 Z2 1:00 Z5 3:00 Z1 2:00 Z4 3:00 Z1 4:00 Z3 3:00 Z1 2:00 Z4	Water, water + electrolytes, or nothing	At least 0.6 g CHO, 0.15 g PRO per kg body weight	

		LEVEL 1 / WEEK 18 / CONTINUED		
	WORKOUT	**NUTRITION DURING WORKOUT**	**RECOVERY NUTRITION (WITHIN 45:00 OF COMPLETING WORKOUT)**	**GENERAL DIET**
T	*Continued* 3:00 Z1 1:00 Z5 3:00 Z1 5:00 Z2 5:00 Z1			4–5 g CHO per kg body weight
W	**Cross-training** Optional			
T	**Foundation run** 5:00 Z1 35:00 Z2 5:00 Z1	Water, water + electrolytes, or nothing	At least 0.4 g CHO, 0.1 g PRO per kg body weight	
F	**Tempo run** 5:00 Z1 7:30 Z2 20:00 Z3 7:30 Z2 5:00 Z1	Water, water + electrolytes, or nothing	At least 0.6 g CHO, 0.15 g PRO per kg body weight	
S	**Cross-training** Optional			
S	**Simulator** 0.5 mile Z1 0.5 mile Z2 26.2 km (16.2 miles) @ marathon race pace	Practice race nutrition plan	At least 1.2 g CHO, 0.3 g PRO per kg body weight	

		LEVEL 1 / WEEK 19		
	WORKOUT	**NUTRITION DURING WORKOUT**	**RECOVERY NUTRITION (WITHIN 45:00 OF COMPLETING WORKOUT)**	**GENERAL DIET**
M	**Rest**			Start 10-day fat-loading period (65 percent of calories from fat) (optional)
T	**Speed-play run** 5:00 Z1 5:00 Z2 1:00 Z5 3:00 Z1 2:00 Z4 3:00 Z1 5:00 Z3 3:00 Z1 2:00 Z4 3:00 Z1 1:00 Z5 3:00 Z1 5:00 Z2 5:00 Z1	Water, water + electrolytes, or nothing	At least 0.6 g CHO, 0.1 g PRO per kg body weight	Day 2 of 10-day fat-loading period (65 percent of calories from fat) (optional)

			LEVEL 1 / WEEK 19 / CONTINUED	
	WORKOUT	**NUTRITION DURING WORKOUT**	**RECOVERY NUTRITION (WITHIN 45:00 OF COMPLETING WORKOUT)**	**GENERAL DIET**
W	**Cross-training** Optional			Day 3 of 10-day fat-loading period (65 percent of calories from fat) (optional)
T	**Foundation run** 5:00 Z1 35:00 Z2 5:00 Z1	Water, water + electrolytes, or nothing	At least 0.4 g CHO, 0.1 g PRO per kg body weight	Day 4 of 10-day fat-loading period (65 percent of calories from fat) (optional)
F	**Tempo run** 5:00 Z1 5:00 Z2 25:00 Z3 5:00 Z2 5:00 Z1	Water, water + electrolytes, or nothing	At least 0.6 g CHO, 0.1 g PRO per kg body weight	Day 5 of 10-day fat-loading period (65 percent of calories from fat) (optional)
S	**Cross-training** Optional			Day 6 of 10-day fat-loading period (65 percent of calories from fat) (optional)
S	**Long run** 0.5 mile Z1 11.0 miles Z2 0.5 mile Z1	Sports drink or gels + water	At least 0.8 g CHO, 0.1 g PRO per kg body weight	Start 7-day caffeine fast (optional) Day 7 of 10-day fat-loading period (65 percent of calories from fat) (optional)

			LEVEL 1 / WEEK 20 / TAPER PERIOD	
	WORKOUT	**NUTRITION DURING WORKOUT**	**RECOVERY NUTRITION (WITHIN 45:00 OF COMPLETING WORKOUT)**	**GENERAL DIET**
M	**Rest**			Reduce caloric intake by amount equal to average per-day reduction in calories burned through training in taper period compared to Week 19 Day 8 of 10-day fat-loading period (65 percent of calories from fat) (optional) OR Start 5-day fat-loading period (optional) Day 2 of 7-day caffeine fast (optional)

	LEVEL 1 / WEEK 20 / TAPER PERIOD / CONTINUED			
	WORKOUT	**NUTRITION DURING WORKOUT**	**RECOVERY NUTRITION (WITHIN 45:00 OF COMPLETING WORKOUT)**	**GENERAL DIET**
T	**Speed-play run** 5:00 Z1 5:00 Z2 6 × (0:30 Z4/ 2:30 Z2) 5:00 Z1	Water, water + electrolytes, or nothing	At least 0.4 g CHO, 0.1 g PRO per kg body weight	Day 2 of reduced calorie intake Day 9 of 10-day fat-loading period (65 percent of calories from fat) (optional) OR Day 2 of 5-day fat-loading period (optional) Day 3 of 7-day caffeine fast (optional)
W	**Cross-training** Optional	Water, water + electrolytes, or nothing	At least 0.4 g CHO, 0.1 g PRO per kg body weight	Day 3 of reduced calorie intake Day 10 of 10-day fat-loading period (65 percent of calories from fat) (optional) OR Day 3 of 5-day fat-loading period (optional) Day 4 of 7-day caffeine fast (optional)
T	**Fast-finish run** 5:00 Z1 20:00 Z2 5:00 Z3	Water, water + electrolytes, or nothing	At least 0.4 g CHO, 0.1 g PRO per kg body weight	Day 4 of reduced calorie intake Day 1 of 3-day carbo-loading period (70 percent of calories from CHO) OR Day 4 of 5-day fat-loading period (optional) Day 5 of 7-day caffeine fast (optional)
F	**Recovery run** 20:00 Z1 OR Cross-training			Day 5 of reduced calorie intake Day 2 of 3-day carbo-loading period (70 percent of calories from CHO) OR Day 5 of 5-day fat-loading period (optional) Day 6 of 7-day caffeine fast (optional)

LEVEL 1 / WEEK 20 / TAPER PERIOD / CONTINUED			
	WORKOUT	NUTRITION DURING WORKOUT	RECOVERY NUTRITION (WITHIN 45:00 OF COMPLETING WORKOUT)	GENERAL DIET

	WORKOUT	NUTRITION DURING WORKOUT	RECOVERY NUTRITION (WITHIN 45:00 OF COMPLETING WORKOUT)	GENERAL DIET
S	Rest			Day 3 of 3-day carbo-loading period (70 percent of calories from CHO) OR Day 1 of 1-day carbo-loading period (10 g CHO per kg body weight) (optional) Day 7 of 7-day caffeine fast (optional)
S	Marathon	Race nutrition plan	Anything you want!	Prerace nutrition plan

LEVEL 2 MARATHON PLAN

Use this twenty-week integrated training and nutrition plan to train for your next marathon if you're ready to work hard to reach the next level but still want to keep your overall training load and time commitment to running manageable. This Level 2 plan includes five runs per week plus one optional cross-training session. You should already be running at least four times per week and up to 6 miles at a time before you start the program.

The training load peaks in Week 18, which includes a marathon Simulator (26.2 km at marathon race pace) and a total of approximately six hours of running. Weeks 4, 8, 12, and 16 are reduced-volume recovery weeks. The program ends with a two-week taper beginning in Week 19.

TABLE 11.2 *LEVEL 2 MARATHON PLAN*

LEVEL 2 / WEEK 1

	WORKOUT	NUTRITION DURING WORKOUT	RECOVERY NUTRITION (WITHIN 45:00 OF COMPLETING WORKOUT)	GENERAL DIET
M	**Rest**			3–4 g CHO per kg body weight
T	**Foundation run** 5:00 Z1 20:00 Z2 5:00 Z1	Water, water + electrolytes, or nothing	At least 0.4 g CHO, 0.1 g PRO per kg body weight	
W	**Foundation run** 5:00 Z1 20:00 Z2 5:00 Z1	Water, water + electrolytes, or nothing	At least 0.4 g CHO, 0.1 g PRO per kg body weight	
T	**Foundation run** 5:00 Z1 20:00 Z2 5:00 Z1	Water, water + electrolytes, or nothing	At least 0.4 g CHO, 0.1 g PRO per kg body weight	
F	**Foundation run** 5:00 Z1 15:00 Z2 5:00 Z1	Water, water + electrolytes, or nothing	At least 0.4 g CHO, 0.1 g PRO per kg body weight	
S	**Cross-training** Optional			
S	**Long run** 0.5 mile Z1 5.0 miles Z2 0.5 mile Z1	Water, water + electrolytes, or nothing	At least 0.4 g CHO, 0.1 g PRO per kg body weight	

LEVEL 2 / WEEK 2

	WORKOUT	NUTRITION DURING WORKOUT	RECOVERY NUTRITION (WITHIN 45:00 OF COMPLETING WORKOUT)	GENERAL DIET
M	**Rest**			3–4 g CHO per kg body weight
T	**Foundation run** 5:00 Z1 25:00 Z2 5:00 Z1	Water, water + electrolytes, or nothing	At least 0.4 g CHO, 0.1 g PRO per kg body weight	
W	**Foundation run** 5:00 Z1 20:00 Z2 5:00 Z1	Water, water + electrolytes, or nothing	At least 0.4 g CHO, 0.1 g PRO per kg body weight	
T	**Foundation run** 5:00 Z1 20:00 Z2 5:00 Z1	Water, water + electrolytes, or nothing	At least 0.4 g CHO, 0.1 g PRO per kg body weight	
F	**Foundation run** 5:00 Z1 25:00 Z2 5:00 Z1	Water, water + electrolytes, or nothing	At least 0.4 g CHO, 0.1 g PRO per kg body weight	

LEVEL 2 / WEEK 2 / CONTINUED

	WORKOUT	NUTRITION DURING WORKOUT	RECOVERY NUTRITION (WITHIN 45:00 OF COMPLETING WORKOUT)	GENERAL DIET
S	**Cross training** Optional			3–4 g CHO per kg body weight
S	**Long run** 0.5 mile Z1 6.0 miles Z2 0.5 mile Z1	Water, water + electrolytes, or nothing	At least 0.4 g CHO, 0.1 g PRO per kg body weight	

LEVEL 2 / WEEK 3

	WORKOUT	NUTRITION DURING WORKOUT	RECOVERY NUTRITION (WITHIN 45:00 OF COMPLETING WORKOUT)	GENERAL DIET
M	**Rest**			3–4 g CHO per kg body weight
T	**Speed-play run** 5:00 Z1 10:00 Z2 6 × (0:15 Z5/ 2:45 Z2) 5:00 Z1	Water, water + electrolytes, or nothing	At least 0.4 g CHO, 0.1 g PRO per kg body weight	
W	**Foundation run** 5:00 Z1 25:00 Z2 5:00 Z1	Water, water + electrolytes, or nothing	At least 0.4 g CHO, 0.1 g PRO per kg body weight	
T	**Foundation run** 5:00 Z1 20:00 Z2 5:00 Z1	Water, water + electrolytes, or nothing	At least 0.4 g CHO, 0.1 g PRO per kg body weight	
F	**Fast-finish run** 5:00 Z1 25:00 Z2 5:00 Z3	Water, water + electrolytes, or nothing	At least 0.4 g CHO, 0.1 g PRO per kg body weight	
S	**Cross training** Optional			
S	**Long run** 0.5 mile Z1 8.0 miles Z2 0.5 mile Z1	Sports drink or gels + water	At least 0.6 g CHO, 0.15 g PRO per kg body weight	

LEVEL 2 / WEEK 4 / RECOVERY WEEK

	WORKOUT	NUTRITION DURING WORKOUT	RECOVERY NUTRITION (WITHIN 45:00 OF COMPLETING WORKOUT)	GENERAL DIET
M	**Rest**			3–4 g CHO per kg body weight
T	**Speed-play run** 5:00 Z1 10:00 Z2 6 × (0:15 Z5/ 2:45 Z2) 5:00 Z1	Water, water + electrolytes, or nothing	At least 0.4 g CHO, 0.1 g PRO per kg body weight	
W	**Foundation run** 5:00 Z1 20:00 Z2 5:00 Z1	Water, water + electrolytes, or nothing	At least 0.4 g CHO, 0.1 g PRO per kg body weight	

LEVEL 2 / WEEK 4 / RECOVERY WEEK / CONTINUED

	WORKOUT	NUTRITION DURING WORKOUT	RECOVERY NUTRITION (WITHIN 45:00 OF COMPLETING WORKOUT)	GENERAL DIET
T	**Foundation run** 5:00 Z1 25:00 Z2 5:00 Z1	Water, water + electrolytes, or nothing	At least 0.4 g CHO, 0.1 g PRO per kg body weight	3–4 g CHO per kg body weight
F	**Fast-finish run** 5:00 Z1 20:00 Z2 5:00 Z3	Water, water + electrolytes, or nothing	At least 0.4 g CHO, 0.1 g PRO per kg body weight	
S	**Cross training** Optional			
S	**Long run** 0.5 mile Z1 7.0 miles Z2 0.5 mile Z1	Water, water + electrolytes, or nothing	At least 0.6 g CHO, 0.15 g PRO per kg body weight	

LEVEL 2 / WEEK 5

	WORKOUT	NUTRITION DURING WORKOUT	RECOVERY NUTRITION (WITHIN 45:00 OF COMPLETING WORKOUT)	GENERAL DIET
M	**Rest**			3–4 g CHO per kg body weight
T	**Hill repetitions run** 5:00 Z1 10:00 Z2 7 × (0:30 Z5/ 2:30 Z1) 5:00 Z1	Water, water + electrolytes, or nothing	At least 0.6 g CHO, 0.1 g PRO per kg body weight	
W	**Foundation run** 5:00 Z1 30:00 Z2 5:00 Z1	Water, water + electrolytes, or nothing	At least 0.4 g CHO, 0.1 g PRO per kg body weight	
T	**Foundation run** 5:00 Z1 30:00 Z2 5:00 Z1	Water, water + electrolytes, or nothing	At least 0.4 g CHO, 0.1 g PRO per kg body weight	
F	**Fast-finish run** 5:00 Z1 30:00 Z2 5:00 Z3	Water, water + electrolytes, or nothing	At least 0.4 g CHO, 0.1 g PRO per kg body weight	
S	**Cross training** Optional			
S	**Long run** 0.5 mile Z1 9.0 miles Z2 0.5 mile Z1	Sports drink or gels + water	At least 0.6 g CHO, 0.15 g PRO per kg body weight	

	LEVEL 2 / WEEK 6			
	WORKOUT	**NUTRITION DURING WORKOUT**	**RECOVERY NUTRITION (WITHIN 45:00 OF COMPLETING WORKOUT)**	**GENERAL DIET**
M	**Rest**			3–4 g CHO per kg body weight
T	**Hill repetitions run** 5:00 Z1 10:00 Z2 9 × (0:30 Z5/ 2:30 Z1) 5:00 Z1	Water, water + electrolytes, or nothing	At least 0.6 g CHO, 0.15 g PRO per kg body weight	
W	**Foundation run** 5:00 Z1 30:00 Z2 5:00 Z1	Water, water + electrolytes, or nothing	At least 0.4 g CHO, 0.1 g PRO per kg body weight	
T	**Foundation run** 5:00 Z1 30:00 Z2 5:00 Z1	Water, water + electrolytes, or nothing	At least 0.4 g CHO, 0.1 g PRO per kg body weight	
F	**Fast-finish run** 5:00 Z1 25:00 Z2 5:00 Z3	Water, water + electrolytes, or nothing	At least 0.4 g CHO, 0.1 g PRO per kg body weight	
S	**Cross training** Optional			
S	**Long run** 0.5 mile Z1 10.0 miles Z2 0.5 mile Z1	Water, water + electrolytes, or nothing	At least 0.6 g CHO, 0.15 g PRO per kg body weight	

	LEVEL 2 / WEEK 7			
	WORKOUT	**NUTRITION DURING WORKOUT**	**RECOVERY NUTRITION (WITHIN 45:00 OF COMPLETING WORKOUT)**	**GENERAL DIET**
M	**Rest**			3–4 g CHO per kg body weight
T	**Hill repetitions run** 5:00 Z1 10:00 Z2 7 × (1:00 Z5/ 2:30 Z1) 5:00 Z1	Water, water + electrolytes, or nothing	At least 0.6 g CHO, 0.15 g PRO per kg body weight	
W	**Foundation run** 5:00 Z1 30:00 Z2 5:00 Z1	Water, water + electrolytes, or nothing	At least 0.4 g CHO, 0.1 g PRO per kg body weight	
T	**Foundation run** 5:00 Z1 30:00 Z2 5:00 Z1	Water, water + electrolytes, or nothing	At least 0.4 g CHO, 0.1 g PRO per kg body weight	
F	**Fast-finish run** 5:00 Z1 25:00 Z2 10:00 Z3	Water, water + electrolytes, or nothing	At least 0.6 g CHO, 0.15 g PRO per kg body weight	

LEVEL 2 / WEEK 7 / CONTINUED				
	WORKOUT	**NUTRITION DURING WORKOUT**	**RECOVERY NUTRITION (WITHIN 45:00 OF COMPLETING WORKOUT)**	**GENERAL DIET**
S	**Cross training** Optional			3–4 g CHO per kg body weight
S	**Long run** 0.5 mile Z1 11.0 miles Z2 0.5 mile Z1	Sports drink or gels + water	At least 0.6 g CHO, 0.15 g PRO per kg body weight	

LEVEL 2 / WEEK 8 / RECOVERY WEEK				
	WORKOUT	**NUTRITION DURING WORKOUT**	**RECOVERY NUTRITION (WITHIN 45:00 OF COMPLETING WORKOUT)**	**GENERAL DIET**
M	**Rest**			3–4 g CHO per kg body weight
T	**Hill repetitions run** 5:00 Z1 10:00 Z2 8 × (0:30 Z5/ 2:30 Z1) 5:00 Z1	Water, water + electrolytes, or nothing	At least 0.6 g CHO, 0.15 g PRO per kg body weight	
W	**Foundation run** 5:00 Z1 25:00 Z2 5:00 Z1	Water, water + electrolytes, or nothing	At least 0.4 g CHO, 0.1 g PRO per kg body weight	
T	**Foundation run** 5:00 Z1 25:00 Z2 5:00 Z1	Water, water + electrolytes, or nothing	At least 0.4 g CHO, 0.1 g PRO per kg body weight	
F	**Fast-finish run** 5:00 Z1 30:00 Z2 10:00 Z3	Water, water + electrolytes, or nothing	At least 0.4 g CHO, 0.1 g PRO per kg body weight	
S	**Cross training** Optional			
S	**Long run** 0.5 mile Z1 9.0 miles Z2 0.5 mile Z1	Water or water + electrolytes	At least 0.6 g CHO, 0.15 g PRO per kg body weight	

LEVEL 2 / WEEK 9				
	WORKOUT	**NUTRITION DURING WORKOUT**	**RECOVERY NUTRITION (WITHIN 45:00 OF COMPLETING WORKOUT)**	**GENERAL DIET**
M	**Rest**			4–5 g CHO per kg body weight
T	**Interval run** 5:00 Z1 10:00 Z2 10 × (1:00 Z5/ 2:00 Z1) 5:00 Z1	Water, water + electrolytes, or nothing	At least 0.8 g CHO, 0.2 g PRO per kg body weight	
W	**Recovery run** 45:00 Z1	Water, water + electrolytes, or nothing	At least 0.4 g CHO, 0.1 g PRO per kg body weight	

LEVEL 2 / WEEK 9 / CONTINUED				
	WORKOUT	NUTRITION DURING WORKOUT	RECOVERY NUTRITION (WITHIN 45:00 OF COMPLETING WORKOUT)	GENERAL DIET
T	**Foundation run** 5:00 Z1 35:00 Z2 5:00 Z1	Water, water + electrolytes, or nothing	At least 0.4 g CHO, 0.1 g PRO per kg body weight	4–5 g CHO per kg body weight
F	**Fast-finish run** 5:00 Z1 25:00 Z2 12:00 Z3	Water, water + electrolytes, or nothing	At least 0.6 g CHO, 0.15 g PRO per kg body weight	
S	**Cross training** Optional			
S	**Long run** 0.5 mile Z1 13.0 miles Z2 0.5 mile Z1	Sports drink or gels + water	At least 0.8 g CHO, 0.2 g PRO per kg body weight	

LEVEL 2 / WEEK 10				
	WORKOUT	NUTRITION DURING WORKOUT	RECOVERY NUTRITION (WITHIN 45:00 OF COMPLETING WORKOUT)	GENERAL DIET
M	Rest			4–5 g CHO per kg body weight
T	**Interval run** 5:00 Z1 10:00 Z2 8 × (1:30 Z5/ 2:30 Z1) 5:00 Z1	Water, water + electrolytes, or nothing	At least 0.6 g CHO, 0.15 g PRO per kg body weight	
W	**Recovery run** 45:00 Z1	Water, water + electrolytes, or nothing	At least 0.4 g CHO, 0.1 g PRO per kg body weight	
T	**Foundation run** 5:00 Z1 35:00 Z2 5:00 Z1	Water, water + electrolytes, or nothing	At least 0.4 g CHO, 0.1 g PRO per kg body weight	
F	**Fast-finish run** 5:00 Z1 28:00 Z2 12:00 Z3	Water, water + electrolytes, or nothing	At least 0.6 g CHO, 0.15 g PRO per kg body weight	
S	**Cross training** Optional			
S	**Long run** 0.5 mile Z1 11.0 miles Z2 0.5 mile Z1	Sports drink or gels + water	At least 0.8 g CHO, 0.2 g PRO per kg body weight	

		LEVEL 2 / WEEK 11		
	WORKOUT	**NUTRITION DURING WORKOUT**	**RECOVERY NUTRITION (WITHIN 45:00 OF COMPLETING WORKOUT)**	**GENERAL DIET**
M	**Rest**			4–5 g CHO per kg body weight
T	**Interval run** 5:00 Z1 10:00 Z2 10 × (1:30 Z5/ 2:30 Z1) 5:00 Z1	Water, water + electrolytes, or nothing	At least 0.8 g CHO, 0.2 g PRO per kg body weight	
W	**Recovery run** 45:00 Z1	Water, water + electrolytes, or nothing	At least 0.4 g CHO, 0.1 g PRO per kg body weight	
T	**Foundation run** 5:00 Z1 35:00 Z2 5:00 Z1	Water, water + electrolytes, or nothing	At least 0.4 g CHO, 0.1 g PRO per kg body weight	
F	**Fast-finish run** 5:00 Z1 33:00 Z2 12:00 Z3	Water, water + electrolytes, or nothing	At least 0.6 g CHO, 0.15 g PRO per kg body weight	
S	**Cross training** Optional			
S	**Long run** 0.5 mile Z1 15.0 miles Z2 0.5 mile Z1	Sports drink or gels + water	At least 1.0 g CHO, 0.25 g PRO per kg body weight	

		LEVEL 2 / WEEK 12 / RECOVERY WEEK		
	WORKOUT	**NUTRITION DURING WORKOUT**	**RECOVERY NUTRITION (WITHIN 45:00 OF COMPLETING WORKOUT)**	**GENERAL DIET**
M	**Rest**			Day 1 of 3-day fat-loading test (optional)
T	**Hill repetitions run** 5:00 Z1 10:00 Z2 8 × (0:30 Z5/ 2:30 Z1) 5:00 Z1	Water, water + electrolytes, or nothing	At least 0.6 g CHO, 0.15 g PRO per kg body weight	Day 2 of 3-day fat-loading test (optional)
W	**Foundation run** 5:00 Z1 30:00 Z2 5:00 Z1	Water, water + electrolytes, or nothing	At least 0.4 g CHO, 0.1 g PRO per kg body weight	Day 3 of 3-day fat-loading test (optional)
T	**Foundation run** 5:00 Z1 30:00 Z2 5:00 Z1	Water, water + electrolytes, or nothing	At least 0.4 g CHO, 0.1 g PRO per kg body weight	4–5 g CHO per kg body weight

LEVEL 2 / WEEK 12 / RECOVERY WEEK / CONTINUED			
	WORKOUT	NUTRITION DURING WORKOUT	RECOVERY NUTRITION (WITHIN 45:00 OF COMPLETING WORKOUT)	GENERAL DIET

	WORKOUT	NUTRITION DURING WORKOUT	RECOVERY NUTRITION (WITHIN 45:00 OF COMPLETING WORKOUT)	GENERAL DIET
F	**Fast-finish run** 5:00 Z1 30:00 Z2 10:00 Z3	Water, water + electrolytes, or nothing	At least 0.4 g CHO, 0.1 g PRO per kg body weight	4–5 g CHO per kg body weight
S	**Cross training** Optional			
S	**Long run** 0.5 mile Z1 10.0 miles Z2 0.5 mile Z1	Water, water + electrolytes, or nothing	At least 0.6 g CHO, 0.15 g PRO per kg body weight	

LEVEL 2 / WEEK 13			

	WORKOUT	NUTRITION DURING WORKOUT	RECOVERY NUTRITION (WITHIN 45:00 OF COMPLETING WORKOUT)	GENERAL DIET
M	**Rest**			4–5 g CHO per kg body weight
T	**Interval run** 5:00 Z1 5:00 Z2 6 × (2:00 Z4/ 2:30 Z1) 5:00 Z1	Water, water + electrolytes, or nothing	At least 0.6 g CHO, 0.15 g PRO per kg body weight	
W	**Recovery run** 40:00 Z1	Water, water + electrolytes, or nothing	At least 0.4 g CHO, 0.1 g PRO per kg body weight	
T	**Foundation run** 5:00 Z1 35:00 Z2 5:00 Z1	Water, water + electrolytes, or nothing	At least 0.4 g CHO, 0.1 g PRO per kg body weight	
F	**Tempo run** 5:00 Z1 10:00 Z2 16:00 Z3 10:00 Z2 5:00 Z1	Water, water + electrolytes, or nothing	At least 0.6 g CHO, 0.15 g PRO per kg body weight	
S	**Cross training** Optional			
S	**Long run** 0.5 mile Z1 17.0 miles Z2 0.5 mile Z1	Sports drink or gels + water	At least 1.0 g CHO, 0.25 g PRO per kg body weight	

LEVEL 2 / WEEK 14			
	WORKOUT	**NUTRITION DURING WORKOUT**	**RECOVERY NUTRITION (WITHIN 45:00 OF COMPLETING WORKOUT)**	**GENERAL DIET**

	WORKOUT	**NUTRITION DURING WORKOUT**	**RECOVERY NUTRITION (WITHIN 45:00 OF COMPLETING WORKOUT)**	**GENERAL DIET**
M	**Rest**			4–5 g CHO per kg body weight
T	**Interval run** 5:00 Z1 5:00 Z2 8 × (2:00 Z4/ 2:30 Z1) 5:00 Z1	Water, water + electrolytes, or nothing	At least 0.8 g CHO, 0.2 g PRO per kg body weight	
W	**Recovery run** 40:00 Z1	Water, water + electrolytes, or nothing	At least 0.4 g CHO, 0.1 g PRO per kg body weight	
T	**Foundation run** 5:00 Z1 35:00 Z2 5:00 Z1	Water, water + electrolytes, or nothing	At least 0.4 g CHO, 0.1 g PRO per kg body weight	
F	**Tempo run** 5:00 Z1 10:00 Z2 20:00 Z3 10:00 Z2 5:00 Z1	Water, water + electrolytes, or nothing	At least 0.6 g CHO, 0.15 g PRO per kg body weight	
S	**Cross training** Optional			
S	**Long run** 0.5 mile Z1 13.0 miles Z2 0.5 mile Z1	Sports drink or gels + water	At least 0.8 g CHO, 0.2 g PRO per kg body weight	

LEVEL 2 / WEEK 15			
	WORKOUT	**NUTRITION DURING WORKOUT**	**RECOVERY NUTRITION (WITHIN 45:00 OF COMPLETING WORKOUT)**	**GENERAL DIET**

	WORKOUT	**NUTRITION DURING WORKOUT**	**RECOVERY NUTRITION (WITHIN 45:00 OF COMPLETING WORKOUT)**	**GENERAL DIET**
M	**Rest**			4–5 g CHO per kg body weight
T	**Interval run** 5:00 Z1 10:00 Z2 5 × (3:00 Z4/ 2:30 Z1) 5:00 Z1	Water, water + electrolytes, or nothing	At least 0.6 g CHO, 0.15 g PRO per kg body weight	
W	**Recovery run** 40:00 Z1	Water, water + electrolytes, or nothing	At least 0.4 g CHO, 0.1 g PRO per kg body weight	
T	**Foundation run** 5:00 Z1 35:00 Z2 5:00 Z1	Water, water + electrolytes, or nothing	At least 0.4 g CHO, 0.1 g PRO per kg body weight	

		NUTRITION DURING WORKOUT	RECOVERY NUTRITION (WITHIN 45:00 OF COMPLETING WORKOUT)	GENERAL DIET
	LEVEL 2 / WEEK 15 / CONTINUED			
	WORKOUT			
F	**Tempo run** 5:00 Z1 10:00 Z2 24:00 Z3 10:00 Z2 5:00 Z1	Water, water + electrolytes, or nothing	At least 0.6 g CHO, 0.15 g PRO per kg body weight	4–5 g CHO per kg body weight
S	**Cross training** Optional			
S	**Long run** 0.5 mile Z1 19.0 miles Z2 0.5 mile Z1	Sports drink or gels + water	At least 1.2 g CHO, 0.3 g PRO per kg body weight	

		NUTRITION DURING WORKOUT	RECOVERY NUTRITION (WITHIN 45:00 OF COMPLETING WORKOUT)	GENERAL DIET
	LEVEL 2 / WEEK 16 / RECOVERY WEEK			
	WORKOUT			
M	**Rest**			4–5 g CHO per kg body weight
T	**Hill repetitions run** 5:00 Z1 10:00 Z2 7 × (1:00 Z5/ 2:30 Z1) 5:00 Z1	Water, water + electrolytes, or nothing	At least 0.6 g CHO, 0.15 g PRO per kg body weight	
W	**Recovery run** 40:00 Z1	Water, water + electrolytes, or nothing	At least 0.4 g CHO, 0.1 g PRO per kg body weight	
T	**Foundation run** 5:00 Z1 30:00 Z2 5:00 Z1	Water, water + electrolytes, or nothing	At least 0.4 g CHO, 0.1 g PRO per kg body weight	
F	**Fast-finish run** 5:00 Z1 25:00 Z2 12:00 Z3	Water, water + electrolytes, or nothing	At least 0.4 g CHO, 0.1 g PRO per kg body weight	
S	**Cross training** Optional			
S	**Long run** 0.5 mile Z1 12.0 miles Z2 0.5 mile Z1	Water, water + electrolytes, or nothing	At least 0.8 g CHO, 0.2 g PRO per kg body weight	

LEVEL 2 / WEEK 17

	WORKOUT	NUTRITION DURING WORKOUT	RECOVERY NUTRITION (WITHIN 45:00 OF COMPLETING WORKOUT)	GENERAL DIET
M	**Rest**			4–5 g CHO per kg body weight
T	**Speed-play run** 5:00 Z1 5:00 Z2 2 × (1:00 Z5/ 2:00 Z1) 2:00 Z4 2:00 Z1 5:00 Z3 2:00 Z1 2:00 Z4 2:00 Z1 2 × (1:00 Z5/ 2:00 Z1) 5:00 Z2 5:00 Z1	Water, water + electrolytes, or nothing	At least 0.6 g CHO, 0.15 g PRO per kg body weight	
W	**Recovery run** 45:00 Z1	Water, water + electrolytes, or nothing	At least 0.4 g CHO, 0.1 g PRO per kg body weight	
T	**Foundation run** 5:00 Z1 35:00 Z2 5:00 Z1	Water, water + electrolytes, or nothing	At least 0.4 g CHO, 0.15 g PRO per kg body weight	
F	**Tempo run** 5:00 Z1 10:00 Z2 28:00 Z3 10:00 Z2 5:00 Z1	Water, water + electrolytes, or nothing	At least 0.8 g CHO, 0.2 g PRO per kg body weight	
S	**Cross training** Optional			
S	**Long run** 0.5 mile Z1 21.0 miles Z2 0.5 mile Z1	Sports drink or gels + water	At least 0.8 g CHO, 0.2 g PRO per kg body weight	

LEVEL 2 / WEEK 18

	WORKOUT	NUTRITION DURING WORKOUT	RECOVERY NUTRITION (WITHIN 45:00 OF COMPLETING WORKOUT)	GENERAL DIET
M	**Rest**			4–5 g CHO per kg body weight
T	**Speed-play run** 5:00 Z1 5:00 Z2 2 × (1:00 Z5/ 2:00 Z1) 2:30 Z4 2:30 Z1	Water, water + electrolytes, or nothing	At least 0.8 g CHO, 0.2 g PRO per kg body weight	

			LEVEL 2 / WEEK 18 / CONTINUED	
	WORKOUT	NUTRITION DURING WORKOUT	RECOVERY NUTRITION (WITHIN 45:00 OF COMPLETING WORKOUT)	GENERAL DIET
T	**Continued** 6:00 Z3 2:00 Z1 2:30 Z4 2:30 Z1 2 × (1:00 Z5/ 2:00 Z1) 5:00 Z2 5:00 Z1			4–5 g CHO per kg body weight
W	**Recovery run** 45:00 Z1	Water, water + electrolytes, or nothing	At least 0.4 g CHO, 0.1 g PRO per kg body weight	
T	**Foundation run** 5:00 Z1 35:00 Z2 5:00 Z1	Water, water + electrolytes, or nothing	At least 0.4 g CHO, 0.1 g PRO per kg body weight	
F	**Tempo run** 5:00 Z1 9:00 Z2 32:00 Z3 9:00 Z2 5:00 Z1	Water, water + electrolytes, or nothing	At least 0.8 g CHO, 0.2 g PRO per kg body weight	
S	**Cross training** Optional			
S	**Simulator** 0.5 mile Z1 0.5 mile Z2 26.2 km (16.2 miles) @ marathon race pace	Practice race nutrition plan	At least 1.2 g CHO, 0.3 g PRO per kg body weight	

			LEVEL 2 / WEEK 19 / TAPER PERIOD	
	WORKOUT	NUTRITION DURING WORKOUT	RECOVERY NUTRITION (WITHIN 45:00 OF COMPLETING WORKOUT)	GENERAL DIET
M	Rest			Reduce caloric intake by amount equal to average per-day reduction in calories burned through training in taper period compared to Week 18 Start 10-day fat-loading period (65 percent of calories from fat) (optional)
T	Speed-play run 5:00 Z1 5:00 Z2 2 × (1:00 Z5/ 2:00 Z1) 2:00 Z4 2:00 Z1 4:00 Z3 2:00 Z1 2:00 Z4 2:00 Z1	Water, water + electrolytes, or nothing	At least 0.6 g CHO, 0.15 g PRO per kg body weight	Day 2 of reduced calorie intake Day 2 of 10-day fat-loading period (65 percent of calories from fat) (optional)

		**LEVEL 2 / WEEK 19 / TAPER PERIOD / CONTINUED**		
	WORKOUT	**NUTRITION DURING WORKOUT**	**RECOVERY NUTRITION (WITHIN 45:00 OF COMPLETING WORKOUT)**	**GENERAL DIET**
T	*Continued* 2 × (1:00 Z5/ 2:00 Z1) 5:00 Z2 5:00 Z1			
W	**Recovery run** 40:00 Z1	Water, water + electrolytes, or nothing	At least 0.4 g CHO, 0.1 g PRO per kg body weight	Day 3 of reduced calorie intake Day 3 of 10-day fat-loading period (65 percent of calories from fat) (optional)
T	**Foundation run** 5:00 Z1 30:00 Z2 5:00 Z1	Water, water + electrolytes, or nothing	At least 0.4 g CHO, 0.1 g PRO per kg body weight	Day 4 of reduced calorie intake Day 4 of 10-day fat-loading period (65 percent of calories from fat) (optional)
F	**Tempo run** 5:00 Z1 5:00 Z2 25:00 Z3 5:00 Z2 5:00 Z1	Water, water + electrolytes, or nothing	At least 0.8 g CHO, 0.2 g PRO per kg body weight	Day 5 of reduced calorie intake Day 5 of 10-day fat-loading period (65 percent of calories from fat) (optional)
S	**Cross training** Optional			Day 6 of reduced calorie intake Day 6 of 10-day fat-loading period (65 percent of calories from fat) (optional)
S	**Long run with fast finish** 0.5 mile Z1 11.5 miles Z2 1.0 mile Z3	Sports drink or gels + water	At least 0.8 g CHO, 0.2 g PRO per kg body weight	Day 7 of reduced calorie intake Start 7-day caffeine fast (optional) Day 7 of 10-day fat-loading period (65 percent of calories from fat) (optional)

		**LEVEL 2 / WEEK 20 / TAPER PERIOD**		
	WORKOUT	**NUTRITION DURING WORKOUT**	**RECOVERY NUTRITION (WITHIN 45:00 OF COMPLETING WORKOUT)**	**GENERAL DIET**
M	**Rest**			Day 8 of reduced calorie intake Day 8 of 10-day fat-loading period (65 percent of calories from fat) (optional) OR Start 5-day fat-loading period (optional) Day 2 of 7-day caffeine fast (optional)

	LEVEL 2 / WEEK 20 / TAPER PERIOD / CONTINUED			
	WORKOUT	NUTRITION DURING WORKOUT	RECOVERY NUTRITION (WITHIN 45:00 OF COMPLETING WORKOUT)	GENERAL DIET
T	**Speed-play run** 5:00 Z1 10:00 Z2 8 × (0:30 Z4/ 2:30 Z2) 5:00 Z1	Water, water + electrolytes, or nothing	At least 0.4 g CHO, 0.1 g PRO per kg body weight	Day 9 of reduced calorie intake Day 9 of 10-day fat-loading period (65 percent of calories from fat) (optional) OR Day 2 of 5-day fat-loading period (optional) Day 3 of 7-day caffeine fast (optional)
W	**Recovery run** 45:00 Z1	Water, water + electrolytes, or nothing	At least 0.4 g CHO, 0.1 g PRO per kg body weight	Day 10 of reduced calorie intake Day 10 of 10-day fat-loading period (65 percent of calories from fat) (optional) OR Day 3 of 5-day fat-loading period (optional) Day 4 of 7-day caffeine fast (optional)
T	**Fast-finish run** 5:00 Z1 20:00 Z2 5:00 Z3	Water, water + electrolytes, or nothing	At least 0.4 g CHO, 0.1 g PRO per kg body weight	Day 11 of reduced calorie intake Day 1 of 3-day carbo-loading period (70 percent of calories from CHO) OR Day 4 of 5-day fat-loading period (optional) Day 5 of 7-day caffeine fast (optional)
F	**Cross-training** Optional			Day 12 of reduced calorie intake Day 2 of 3-day carbo-loading period (70 percent of calories from CHO) OR Day 5 of 5-day fat-loading period (optional) Day 6 of 7-day caffeine fast (optional)
S	**Speed-play run** 5:00 Z1 5:00 Z2 4 × (0:30 Z4/ 1:30 Z2) 5:00 Z1	Water, water + electrolytes, or nothing	At least 0.4 g CHO, 0.1 g PRO per kg body weight	Day 3 of 3-day carbo-loading period (70 percent of calories from CHO) OR Day 1 of 1-day carbo-loading period (10 g CHO per kg body weight) (optional) Day 7 of 7-day caffeine fast (optional)
S	**Marathon**	Race nutrition plan	Anything you want!	Prerace nutrition plan

LEVEL 3 MARATHON PLAN

The workload in this twenty-week integrated training and nutrition plan is about as heavy as any runner preparing for a marathon can sensibly take on without training twice a day. It includes either seven runs or, optionally, six runs and one cross-training per week in most weeks. You should already be running more or less daily and be able to comfortably go at least 8 miles before you start the program.

The most challenging week of the program is Week 18, which includes a marathon Simulator (26.2 km at marathon race pace) and a total of approximately eight hours of running. Weeks 4, 7, 10, 13, and 16 are reduced-volume recovery weeks. There is a two-week taper starting at Week 19.

TABLE 11.3 *LEVEL 3 MARATHON PLAN*				
LEVEL 3 / WEEK 1				
	WORKOUT	NUTRITION DURING WORKOUT	RECOVERY NUTRITION (WITHIN 45:00 OF COMPLETING WORKOUT)	GENERAL DIET
M	Rest			4–5 g CHO per kg body weight
T	**Foundation run** 5:00 Z1 30:00 Z2 5:00 Z1 OR Cross-training	Water, water + electrolytes, or nothing	At least 0.4 g CHO, 0.1 g PRO per kg body weight	
W	**Foundation run** 5:00 Z1 30:00 Z2 5:00 Z1	Water, water + electrolytes, or nothing	At least 0.4 g CHO, 0.1 g PRO per kg body weight	
T	**Foundation run** 5:00 Z1 30:00 Z2 5:00 Z1	Water, water + electrolytes, or nothing	At least 0.4 g CHO, 0.1 g PRO per kg body weight	
F	**Foundation run** 5:00 Z1 30:00 Z2 5:00 Z1	Water, water + electrolytes, or nothing	At least 0.4 g CHO, 0.1 g PRO per kg body weight	
S	**Foundation run** 5:00 Z1 30:00 Z2 5:00 Z1	Water, water + electrolytes, or nothing	At least 0.4 g CHO, 0.1 g PRO per kg body weight	
S	**Long run** 0.5 mile Z1 7.0 miles Z2 0.5 mile Z1	Water, water + electrolytes, or nothing	At least 0.6 g CHO, 0.15 g PRO per kg body weight	

	WORKOUT	NUTRITION DURING WORKOUT	RECOVERY NUTRITION (WITHIN 45:00 OF COMPLETING WORKOUT)	GENERAL DIET
			LEVEL 3 / WEEK 2	
M	**Foundation run** 5:00 Z1 35:00 Z2 5:00 Z1 OR Cross-training	Water, water + electrolytes, or nothing	At least 0.4 g CHO, 0.1 g PRO per kg body weight	4–5 g CHO per kg body weight
T	**Speed-play run** 5:00 Z1 10:00 Z2 10 × (0:15 Z5/ 2:45 Z2) 5:00 Z1	Water, water + electrolytes, or nothing	At least 0.4 g CHO, 0.1 g PRO per kg body weight	
W	**Foundation run** 5:00 Z1 35:00 Z2 5:00 Z1	Water, water + electrolytes, or nothing	At least 0.4 g CHO, 0.1 g PRO per kg body weight	
T	**Foundation run** 5:00 Z1 35:00 Z2 5:00 Z1	Water, water + electrolytes, or nothing	At least 0.4 g CHO, 0.1 g PRO per kg body weight	
F	**Foundation run** 5:00 Z1 35:00 Z2 5:00 Z1	Water, water + electrolytes, or nothing	At least 0.4 g CHO, 0.1 g PRO per kg body weight	
S	**Foundation run** 5:00 Z1 35:00 Z2 5:00 Z1	Water, water + electrolytes, or nothing	At least 0.4 g CHO, 0.1 g PRO per kg body weight	
S	**Long run** 0.5 mile Z1 8.0 miles Z2 0.5 mile Z1	Water, water + electrolytes, or nothing	At least 0.6 g CHO, 0.15 g PRO per kg body weight	

	WORKOUT	NUTRITION DURING WORKOUT	RECOVERY NUTRITION (WITHIN 45:00 OF COMPLETING WORKOUT)	GENERAL DIET
			LEVEL 3 / WEEK 3	
M	**Foundation run** 5:00 Z1 35:00 Z2 5:00 Z1 OR Cross-training	Water, water + electrolytes, or nothing	At least 0.4 g CHO, 0.1 g PRO per kg body weight	4–5 g CHO per kg body weight
T	**Speed-play run** 5:00 Z1 10:00 Z2 10 × (0:30 Z5/ 2:30 Z2) 5:00 Z1	Water, water + electrolytes, or nothing	At least 0.6 g CHO, 0.15 g PRO per kg body weight	
W	**Foundation run** 5:00 Z1 35:00 Z2 5:00 Z1	Water, water + electrolytes, or nothing	At least 0.4 g CHO, 0.1 g PRO per kg body weight	

LEVEL 3 / WEEK 3 / CONTINUED				
	WORKOUT	NUTRITION DURING WORKOUT	RECOVERY NUTRITION (WITHIN 45:00 OF COMPLETING WORKOUT)	GENERAL DIET
T	**Foundation run** 5:00 Z1 35:00 Z2 5:00 Z1	Water, water + electrolytes, or nothing	At least 0.4 g CHO, 0.1 g PRO per kg body weight	4–5 g CHO per kg body weight
F	**Fast-finish run** 5:00 Z1 40:00 Z2 5:00 Z3	Water, water + electrolytes, or nothing	At least 0.6 g CHO, 0.15 g PRO per kg body weight	
S	**Foundation run** 5:00 Z1 35:00 Z2 5:00 Z1	Water, water + electrolytes, or nothing	At least 0.4 g CHO, 0.1 g PRO per kg body weight	
S	**Long run** 0.5 mile Z1 9.0 miles Z2 0.5 mile Z1	Water, water + electrolytes, or nothing	At least 0.6 g CHO, 0.15 g PRO per kg body weight	

LEVEL 3 / WEEK 4 / RECOVERY WEEK				
	WORKOUT	NUTRITION DURING WORKOUT	RECOVERY NUTRITION (WITHIN 45:00 OF COMPLETING WORKOUT)	GENERAL DIET
M	**Rest**			4–5 g CHO per kg body weight
T	**Hill repetitions run** 5:00 Z1 10:00 Z2 10 × (0:30 Z5/ 2:30 Z1) 5:00 Z1	Water, water + electrolytes, or nothing	At least 0.8 g CHO, 0.2 g PRO per kg body weight	
W	**Recovery run** 45:00 Z1	Water, water + electrolytes, or nothing	At least 0.4 g CHO, 0.1 g PRO per kg body weight	
T	**Foundation run** 5:00 Z1 35:00 Z2 5:00 Z1	Water, water + electrolytes, or nothing	At least 0.4 g CHO, 0.1 g PRO per kg body weight	
F	**Fast-finish run** 5:00 Z1 40:00 Z2 5:00 Z3	Water, water + electrolytes, or nothing	At least 0.6 g CHO, 0.15 g PRO per kg body weight	
S	**Foundation run** 5:00 Z1 30:00 Z2 5:00 Z1	Water, water + electrolytes, or nothing	At least 0.4 g CHO, 0.1 g PRO per kg body weight	
S	**Long run** 0.5 mile Z1 7.0 miles Z2 0.5 mile Z1	Sports drink or gels + water	At least 0.6 g CHO, 0.15 g PRO per kg body weight	

			LEVEL 3 / WEEK 5	
	WORKOUT	**NUTRITION DURING WORKOUT**	**RECOVERY NUTRITION (WITHIN 45:00 OF COMPLETING WORKOUT)**	**GENERAL DIET**
M	**Foundation run** 5:00 Z1 40:00 Z2 5:00 Z1	Water, water + electrolytes, or nothing	At least 0.4 g CHO, 0.1 g PRO per kg body weight	5–6 g CHO per kg body weight
T	**Hill repetitions run** 5:00 Z1 10:00 Z2 14 × (0:30 Z5/ 2:30 Z1) 5:00 Z1	Water, water + electrolytes, or nothing	At least 0.8 g CHO, 0.2 g PRO per kg body weight	
W	**Recovery run** 45:00 Z1	Water, water + electrolytes, or nothing	At least 0.4 g CHO, 0.1 g PRO per kg body weight	
T	**Foundation run** 5:00 Z1 40:00 Z2 5:00 Z1	Water, water + electrolytes, or nothing	At least 0.4 g CHO, 0.1 g PRO per kg body weight	
F	**Fast-finish run** 5:00 Z1 35:00 Z2 10:00 Z3	Water, water + electrolytes, or nothing	At least 0.6 g CHO, 0.15 g PRO per kg body weight	
S	**Foundation run** 5:00 Z1 40:00 Z2 5:00 Z1	Water, water + electrolytes, or nothing	At least 0.4 g CHO, 0.1 g PRO per kg body weight	
S	**Long run** 0.5 mile Z1 11.0 miles Z2 0.5 mile Z1	Sports drink or gels + water	At least 0.8 g CHO, 0.2 g PRO per kg body weight	

			LEVEL 3 / WEEK 6	
	WORKOUT	**NUTRITION DURING WORKOUT**	**RECOVERY NUTRITION (WITHIN 45:00 OF COMPLETING WORKOUT)**	**GENERAL DIET**
M	**Foundation run** 5:00 Z1 40:00 Z2 5:00 Z1 OR Cross-training	Water, water + electrolytes, or nothing	At least 0.4 g CHO, 0.1 g PRO per kg body weight	5–6 g CHO per kg body weight
T	**Hill repetitions run** 5:00 Z1 10:00 Z2 12 × (1:00 Z5/ 2:30 Z1) 5:00 Z1	Sports drink or gels + water	At least 0.8 g CHO, 0.2 g PRO per kg body weight	
W	**Recovery run** 45:00 Z1	Water, water + electrolytes, or nothing	At least 0.4 g CHO, 0.1 g PRO per kg body weight	

LEVEL 3 / WEEK 6 / CONTINUED

	WORKOUT	NUTRITION DURING WORKOUT	RECOVERY NUTRITION (WITHIN 45:00 OF COMPLETING WORKOUT)	GENERAL DIET
T	**Foundation run** 5:00 Z1 40:00 Z2 5:00 Z1	Water, water + electrolytes, or nothing	At least 0.6 g CHO, 0.15 g PRO per kg body weight	5–6 g CHO per kg body weight
F	**Fast-finish run** 5:00 Z1 45:00 Z2 10:00 Z3	Water, water + electrolytes, or nothing	At least 0.8 g CHO, 0.2 g PRO per kg body weight	
S	**Foundation run** 5:00 Z1 40:00 Z2 5:00 Z1	Water, water + electrolytes, or nothing	At least 0.6 g CHO, 0.12 g PRO per kg body weight	
S	**Long run** 0.5 mile Z1 12.0 miles Z2 0.5 mile Z1	Water, water + electrolytes, or nothing	At least 0.8 g CHO, 0.2 g PRO per kg body weight	

LEVEL 3 / WEEK 7 / RECOVERY WEEK

	WORKOUT	NUTRITION DURING WORKOUT	RECOVERY NUTRITION (WITHIN 45:00 OF COMPLETING WORKOUT)	GENERAL DIET
M	**Rest**			5–6 g CHO per kg body weight
T	**Hill repetitions run** 5:00 Z1 10:00 Z2 8 × (1:00 Z5/ 2:30 Z1) 5:00 Z1	Sports drink or gels + water	At least 0.8 g CHO, 0.2 g PRO per kg body weight	
W	**Recovery run** 45:00 Z1	Water, water + electrolytes, or nothing	At least 0.4 g CHO, 0.1 g PRO per kg body weight	
T	**Foundation run** 5:00 Z1 40:00 Z2 5:00 Z1	Water, water + electrolytes, or nothing	At least 0.6 g CHO, 0.15 g PRO per kg body weight	
F	**Fast-finish run** 5:00 Z1 40:00 Z2 10:00 Z3	Water, water + electrolytes, or nothing	At least 0.8 g CHO, 0.2 g PRO per kg body weight	
S	**Foundation run** 5:00 Z1 40:00 Z2 5:00 Z1	Water, water + electrolytes, or nothing	At least 0.6 g CHO, 0.12 g PRO per kg body weight	
S	**Long run** 0.5 mile Z1 10.0 miles Z2 0.5 mile Z1	Water, water + electrolytes, or nothing	At least 0.8 g CHO, 0.2 g PRO per kg body weight	

LEVEL 3 / WEEK 8				
	WORKOUT	NUTRITION DURING WORKOUT	RECOVERY NUTRITION (WITHIN 45:00 OF COMPLETING WORKOUT)	GENERAL DIET
M	**Foundation run** 5:00 Z1 40:00 Z2 5:00 Z1	Water, water + electrolytes, or nothing	At least 0.4 g CHO, 0.1 g PRO per kg body weight	5–6 g CHO per kg body weight
T	**Hill repetitions run** 5:00 Z1 10:00 Z2 12 × (1:00 Z5/ 2:30 Z1) 5:00 Z1	Sports drink or gels + water	At least 0.8 g CHO, 0.2 g PRO per kg body weight	
W	**Recovery run** 45:00 Z1	Water, water + electrolytes, or nothing	At least 0.4 g CHO, 0.1 g PRO per kg body weight	
T	**Foundation run** 5:00 Z1 40:00 Z2 5:00 Z1	Water, water + electrolytes, or nothing	At least 0.6 g CHO, 0.15 g PRO per kg body weight	
F	**Fast-finish run** 5:00 Z1 50:00 Z2 10:00 Z3	Water, water + electrolytes, or nothing	At least 0.8 g CHO, 0.2 g PRO per kg body weight	
S	**Foundation run** 5:00 Z1 40:00 Z2 5:00 Z1	Water, water + electrolytes, or nothing	At least 0.6 g CHO, 0.12 g PRO per kg body weight	
S	**Long run** 0.5 mile Z1 12.0 miles Z2 0.5 mile Z1	Water or water + electrolytes	At least 0.8 g CHO, 0.2 g PRO per kg body weight	

LEVEL 3 / WEEK 9				
	WORKOUT	NUTRITION DURING WORKOUT	RECOVERY NUTRITION (WITHIN 45:00 OF COMPLETING WORKOUT)	GENERAL DIET
M	**Foundation run** 5:00 Z1 35:00 Z2 5:00 Z1 OR Cross-training	Water, water + electrolytes, or nothing	At least 0.4 g CHO, 0.1 g PRO per kg body weight	5–6 g CHO per kg body weight
T	**Interval run** 5:00 Z1 5:00 Z2 12 × (1:00 Z5/ 2:30 Z1) 5:00 Z1	Sports drink or gels + water	At least 0.8 g CHO, 0.2 g PRO per kg body weight	
W	**Recovery run** 45:00 Z1	Water, water + electrolytes, or nothing	At least 0.4 g CHO, 0.1 g PRO per kg body weight	

	LEVEL 3 / WEEK 9 / CONTINUED			
	WORKOUT	NUTRITION DURING WORKOUT	RECOVERY NUTRITION (WITHIN 45:00 OF COMPLETING WORKOUT)	GENERAL DIET
T	**Foundation run** 5:00 Z1 35:00 Z2 5:00 Z1	Water, water + electrolytes, or nothing	At least 0.4 g CHO, 0.1 g PRO per kg body weight	5–6 g CHO per kg body weight
F	**Fast-finish run** 5:00 Z1 40:00 Z2 15:00 Z3	Water, water + electrolytes, or nothing	At least 0.8 g CHO, 0.2 g PRO per kg body weight	
S	**Foundation run** 5:00 Z1 35:00 Z2 5:00 Z1	Water, water + electrolytes, or nothing	At least 0.4 g CHO, 0.1 g PRO per kg body weight	
S	**Long run** 0.5 mile Z1 13.0 miles Z2 0.5 mile Z1	Sports drink or gels + water	At least 0.8 g CHO, 0.2 g PRO per kg body weight	

	LEVEL 3 / WEEK 10 / RECOVERY WEEK			
	WORKOUT	NUTRITION DURING WORKOUT	RECOVERY NUTRITION (WITHIN 45:00 OF COMPLETING WORKOUT)	GENERAL DIET
M	**Foundation run** 5:00 Z1 35:00 Z2 5:00 Z1 OR Cross-training	Water, water + electrolytes, or nothing	At least 0.4 g CHO, 0.1 g PRO per kg body weight	5–6 g CHO per kg body weight
T	**Interval run** 5:00 Z1 5:00 Z2 9 × (1:00 Z5/ 2:30 Z1) 5:00 Z1	Sports drink or gels + water	At least 0.8 g CHO, 0.2 g PRO per kg body weight	
W	**Recovery run** 45:00 Z1	Water, water + electrolytes, or nothing	At least 0.4 g CHO, 0.1 g PRO per kg body weight	
T	**Foundation run** 5:00 Z1 35:00 Z2 5:00 Z1	Water, water + electrolytes, or nothing	At least 0.4 g CHO, 0.1 g PRO per kg body weight	
F	**Fast-finish run** 5:00 Z1 45:00 Z2 10:00 Z3	Water, water + electrolytes, or nothing	At least 0.8 g CHO, 0.2 g PRO per kg body weight	
S	**Foundation run** 5:00 Z1 35:00 Z2 5:00 Z1	Water, water + electrolytes, or nothing	At least 0.4 g CHO, 0.1 g PRO per kg body weight	
S	**Long run** 0.5 mile Z1 10.0 miles Z2 0.5 mile Z1	Water or water + electrolytes	At least 0.8 g CHO, 0.2 g PRO per kg body weight	

			LEVEL 3 / WEEK 11	
	WORKOUT	**NUTRITION DURING WORKOUT**	**RECOVERY NUTRITION (WITHIN 45:00 OF COMPLETING WORKOUT)**	**GENERAL DIET**
M	**Foundation run** 5:00 Z1 40:00 Z2 5:00 Z1 OR Cross-training	Water, water + electrolytes, or nothing	At least 0.4 g CHO, 0.1 g PRO per kg body weight	5–6 g CHO per kg body weight
T	**Interval run** 5:00 Z1 5:00 Z2 10 × (1:30 Z5/ 2:30 Z1) 5:00 Z1	Water or water + electrolytes	At least 0.8 g CHO, 0.2 g PRO per kg body weight	
W	**Recovery run** 45:00 Z1	Water, water + electrolytes, or nothing	At least 0.4 g CHO, 0.1 g PRO per kg body weight	
T	**Foundation run** 5:00 Z1 40:00 Z2 5:00 Z1	Water, water + electrolytes, or nothing	At least 0.4 g CHO, 0.1 g PRO per kg body weight	
F	**Fast-finish run** 5:00 Z1 45:00 Z2 15:00 Z3	Water, water + electrolytes, or nothing	At least 0.8 g CHO, 0.2 g PRO per kg body weight	
S	**Foundation run** 5:00 Z1 40:00 Z2 5:00 Z1	Water, water + electrolytes, or nothing	At least 0.4 g CHO, 0.1 g PRO per kg body weight	
S	**Long run** 0.5 mile Z1 15.0 miles Z2 0.5 mile Z1	Sports drink or gels + water	At least 1.0 g CHO, 0.25 g PRO per kg body weight	

			LEVEL 3 / WEEK 12	
	WORKOUT	**NUTRITION DURING WORKOUT**	**RECOVERY NUTRITION (WITHIN 45:00 OF COMPLETING WORKOUT)**	**GENERAL DIET**
M	**Recovery run** 50:00 Z1 OR Cross-training	Water, water + electrolytes, or nothing	At least 0.4 g CHO, 0.1 g PRO per kg body weight	5–6 g CHO per kg body weight
T	**Interval run** 5:00 Z1 5:00 Z2 12 × (1:30 Z5/ 2:30 Z1) 5:00 Z1	Sports drink or gels + water	At least 0.8 g CHO, 0.2 g PRO per kg body weight	
W	**Recovery run** 50:00 Z1	Water, water + electrolytes, or nothing	At least 0.4 g CHO, 0.1 g PRO per kg body weight	

	WORKOUT	NUTRITION DURING WORKOUT	RECOVERY NUTRITION (WITHIN 45:00 OF COMPLETING WORKOUT)	GENERAL DIET
	**LEVEL 3 / WEEK 12 / CONTINUED**			
T	**Foundation run** 5:00 Z1 40:00 Z2 5:00 Z1	Water, water + electrolytes, or nothing	At least 0.4 g CHO, 0.1 g PRO per kg body weight	5–6 g CHO per kg body weight
F	**Tempo run** 5:00 Z1 10:00 Z2 20:00 Z3 10:00 Z2 5:00 Z1	Water, water + electrolytes, or nothing	At least 0.6 g CHO, 0.15 g PRO per kg body weight	
S	**Foundation run** 5:00 Z1 40:00 Z2 5:00 Z1	Water, water + electrolytes, or nothing	At least 0.4 g CHO, 0.1 g PRO per kg body weight	
S	**Long run** 0.5 mile Z1 17.0 miles Z2 0.5 mile Z1	Sports drink or gels + water	At least 1.0 g CHO, 0.25 g PRO per kg body weight	

	WORKOUT	NUTRITION DURING WORKOUT	RECOVERY NUTRITION (WITHIN 45:00 OF COMPLETING WORKOUT)	GENERAL DIET
	**LEVEL 3 / WEEK 13 / RECOVERY WEEK**			
M	**Rest**			Day 1 of 3-day fat-loading test (optional)
T	**Interval run** 5:00 Z1 10:00 Z2 7 × (2:00 Z4/ 2:30 Z1) 5:00 Z1	Water, water + electrolytes, or nothing	At least 0.8 g CHO, 0.2 g PRO per kg body weight	Day 2 of 3-day fat-loading test (optional)
W	**Recovery run** 45:00 Z1	Water, water + electrolytes, or nothing	At least 0.4 g CHO, 0.1 g PRO per kg body weight	Day 3 of 3-day fat-loading test (optional)
T	**Foundation run** 5:00 Z1 40:00 Z2 5:00 Z1	Water, water + electrolytes, or nothing	At least 0.6 g CHO, 0.15 g PRO per kg body weight	5–6 g CHO per kg body weight
F	**Fast-finish run** 5:00 Z1 30:00 Z2 15:00 Z3	Water, water + electrolytes, or nothing	At least 0.6 g CHO, 0.15 g PRO per kg body weight	
S	**Recovery run** 50:00 Z1	Water, water + electrolytes, or nothing	At least 0.6 g CHO, 0.15 g PRO per kg body weight	
S	**Long run** 0.5 mile Z1 12.0 miles Z2 0.5 mile Z1	Water, water + electrolytes, or nothing	At least 0.8 g CHO, 0.2 g PRO per kg body weight	

	LEVEL 3 / WEEK 14			
	WORKOUT	NUTRITION DURING WORKOUT	RECOVERY NUTRITION (WITHIN 45:00 OF COMPLETING WORKOUT)	GENERAL DIET
M	**Recovery run** 55:00 Z1 OR Cross-training	Water, water + electrolytes, or nothing	At least 0.8 g CHO, 0.2 g PRO per kg body weight	5–6 g CHO per kg body weight
T	**Interval run** 5:00 Z1 10:00 Z2 9 × (2:00 Z4/ 2:30 Z1) 5:00 Z1	Water or water + electrolytes	At least 0.8 g CHO, 0.2 g PRO per kg body weight	
W	**Recovery run** 50:00 Z1	Water, water + electrolytes, or nothing	At least 0.4 g CHO, 0.1 g PRO per kg body weight	
T	**Foundation run** 5:00 Z1 50:00 Z2 5:00 Z1	Water, water + electrolytes, or nothing	At least 0.6 g CHO, 0.15 g PRO per kg body weight	
F	**Tempo run** 5:00 Z1 10:00 Z2 28:00 Z3 10:00 Z2 5:00 Z1	Water, water + electrolytes, or nothing	At least 0.8 g CHO, 0.2 g PRO per kg body weight	
S	**Foundation run** 5:00 Z1 45:00 Z2 5:00 Z1	Water, water + electrolytes, or nothing	At least 0.6 g CHO, 0.15 g PRO per kg body weight	
S	**Long run** 0.5 mile Z1 19.0 miles Z2 0.5 mile Z1	Sports drink or gels + water	At least 1.2 g CHO, 0.3 g PRO per kg body weight	

	LEVEL 3 / WEEK 15			
	WORKOUT	NUTRITION DURING WORKOUT	RECOVERY NUTRITION (WITHIN 45:00 OF COMPLETING WORKOUT)	GENERAL DIET
M	**Foundation run** 5:00 Z1 45:00 Z2 5:00 Z1 OR Cross-training	Water, water + electrolytes, or nothing	At least 0.6 g CHO, 0.15 g PRO per kg body weight	5–6 g CHO per kg body weight
T	**Interval run** 5:00 Z1 10:00 Z2 6 × (3:00 Z4/ 2:30 Z1) 5:00 Z1	Water, water + electrolytes, or nothing	At least 0.8 g CHO, 0.2 g PRO per kg body weight	
W	**Recovery run** 50:00 Z1	Water, water + electrolytes, or nothing	At least 0.4 g CHO, 0.1 g PRO per kg body weight	

	WORKOUT	NUTRITION DURING WORKOUT	RECOVERY NUTRITION (WITHIN 45:00 OF COMPLETING WORKOUT)	GENERAL DIET
	LEVEL 3 / WEEK 15 / CONTINUED			
T	**Foundation run** 5:00 Z1 45:00 Z2 5:00 Z1	Water, water + electrolytes, or nothing	At least 0.6 g CHO, 0.15 g PRO per kg body weight	5–6 g CHO per kg body weight
F	**Tempo run** 5:00 Z1 10:00 Z2 32:00 Z3 10:00 Z2 5:00 Z1	Sports drink or gels + water	At least 0.8 g CHO, 0.2 g PRO per kg body weight	
S	**Recovery run** 50:00 Z1	Water, water + electrolytes, or nothing	At least 0.4 g CHO, 0.1 g PRO per kg body weight	
S	**Long run** 0.5 mile Z1 21.0 miles Z2 0.5 mile Z1	Sports drink or gels + water	At least 1.2 g CHO, 0.3 g PRO per kg body weight	

	WORKOUT	NUTRITION DURING WORKOUT	RECOVERY NUTRITION (WITHIN 45:00 OF COMPLETING WORKOUT)	GENERAL DIET
	LEVEL 3 / WEEK 16 / RECOVERY WEEK			
M	**Rest**			5–6 g CHO per kg body weight
T	**Hill repetitions run** 5:00 Z1 10:00 Z2 8 × (1:00 Z5/ 2:30 Z1) 5:00 Z1	Water, water + electrolytes, or nothing	At least 0.6 g CHO, 0.15 g PRO per kg body weight	
W	**Recovery run** 50:00 Z1	Water, water + electrolytes, or nothing	At least 0.4 g CHO, 0.1 g PRO per kg body weight	
T	**Foundation run** 5:00 Z1 35:00 Z2 5:00 Z1	Water, water + electrolytes, or nothing	At least 0.4 g CHO, 0.1 g PRO per kg body weight	
F	**Tempo run** 5:00 Z1 10:00 Z2 20:00 Z3 10:00 Z2 5:00 Z1	Water, water + electrolytes, or nothing	At least 0.8 g CHO, 0.2 g PRO per kg body weight	
S	**Foundation run** 5:00 Z1 35:00 Z2 5:00 Z1	Water, water + electrolytes, or nothing	At least 0.4 g CHO, 0.1 g PRO per kg body weight	
S	**Long run with fast finish** 0.5 mile Z1 12.5 miles Z2 1.0 mile Z3	Water, water + electrolytes, or nothing	At least 0.8 g CHO, 0.2 g PRO per kg body weight	

	LEVEL 3 / WEEK 17			
	WORKOUT	**NUTRITION DURING WORKOUT**	**RECOVERY NUTRITION (WITHIN 45:00 OF COMPLETING WORKOUT)**	**GENERAL DIET**
M	**Foundation run** 5:00 Z1 50:00 Z2 5:00 Z1 OR Cross-training	Water, water + electrolytes, or nothing	At least 0.6 g CHO, 0.15 g PRO per kg body weight	6–7 g CHO per kg body weight
T	**Interval run** 5:00 Z1 10:00 Z2 5 × (4:00 Z4/ 2:30 Z1) 5:00 Z1	Water or water + electrolytes	At least 0.8 g CHO, 0.2 g PRO per kg body weight	
W	**Recovery run** 60:00 Z1	Water, water + electrolytes, or nothing	At least 0.6 g CHO, 0.15 g PRO per kg body weight	
T	**Foundation run** 5:00 Z1 50:00 Z2 5:00 Z1	Water, water + electrolytes, or nothing	At least 0.6 g CHO, 0.15 g PRO per kg body weight	
F	**Tempo run** 5:00 Z1 10:00 Z2 36:00 Z3 10:00 Z2 5:00 Z1	Water, water + electrolytes, or nothing	At least 0.8 g CHO, 0.2 g PRO per kg body weight	
S	**Recovery run** 60:00 Z1	Water, water + electrolytes, or nothing	At least 0.6 g CHO, 0.15 g PRO per kg body weight	
S	**Long run with fast finish** 0.5 mile Z1 22.5 miles Z2 1 mile Z3	Sports drink or gels + water	At least 1.2 g CHO, 0.3 g PRO per kg body weight	

	LEVEL 3 / WEEK 18			
	WORKOUT	**NUTRITION DURING WORKOUT**	**RECOVERY NUTRITION (WITHIN 45:00 OF COMPLETING WORKOUT)**	**GENERAL DIET**
M	**Recovery run** 60:00 Z1	Water, water + electrolytes, or nothing	At least 0.6 g CHO, 0.15 g PRO per kg body weight	6–7 g CHO per kg body weight
T	**Speed-play run** 5:00 Z1 5:00 Z2 2 × (1:00 Z2/2:00 Z1) 2 × (2:30 Z4/2:30 Z1) 6:00 Z3	Water, water + electrolytes, or nothing	At least 0.8 g CHO, 0.2 g PRO per kg body weight	

LEVEL 3 / WEEK 18 / CONTINUED			
	WORKOUT	NUTRITION DURING WORKOUT	RECOVERY NUTRITION (WITHIN 45:00 OF COMPLETING WORKOUT)	GENERAL DIET
T	**Continued** 2:00 Z1 2 × (2:30 Z4/2:30 Z1) 2 × (1:00 Z2/2:00 Z1) 5:00 Z2 5:00 Z1			6–7 g CHO per kg body weight
W	**Recovery run** 60:00 Z1	Water, water + electrolytes, or nothing	At least 0.4 g CHO, 0.1 g PRO per kg body weight	
T	**Foundation run** 5:00 Z1 40:00 Z2 5:00 Z1	Water, water + electrolytes, or nothing	At least 0.4 g CHO, 0.1 g PRO per kg body weight	
F	**Tempo run** 5:00 Z1 10:00 Z2 40:00 Z3 10:00 Z2 5:00 Z1	Sports drink or gels + water	At least 0.8 g CHO, 0.2 g PRO per kg body weight	
S	**Recovery run** 60:00 Z1	Water, water + electrolytes, or nothing	At least 0.6 g CHO, 0.15 g PRO per kg body weight	
S	**Simulator** 0.5 mile Z1 0.5 mile Z2 26.2 km (16.2 miles) @ marathon race pace	Prerace nutrition plan	At least 1.2 g CHO, 0.3 g PRO per kg body weight	

LEVEL 3 / WEEK 19 / TAPER PERIOD			
	WORKOUT	NUTRITION DURING WORKOUT	RECOVERY NUTRITION (WITHIN 45:00 OF COMPLETING WORKOUT)	GENERAL DIET
M	Rest			Reduce caloric intake by amount equal to average per-day reduction in calories burned through training in taper period compared to Week 18 Start 10-day fat-loading period (65 percent of calories from fat) (optional)
T	**Interval run** 5:00 Z1 5:00 Z2 2 × (1:00 Z5/2:00 Z1) 2:00 Z4 2:00 Z1 5:00 Z3 2:00 Z1	Water, water + electrolytes, or nothing	At least 0.6 g CHO, 0.15 g PRO per kg body weight	Day 2 of reduced calorie intake Day 2 of 10-day fat-loading period (65 percent of calories from fat) (optional)

	LEVEL 3 / WEEK 19 / TAPER PERIOD / CONTINUED			
	WORKOUT	**NUTRITION DURING WORKOUT**	**RECOVERY NUTRITION (WITHIN 45:00 OF COMPLETING WORKOUT)**	**GENERAL DIET**
T	*Continued* 2:00 Z4 2:00 Z1 2 × (1:00 Z5/ 2:00 Z1) 5:00 Z2 5:00 Z1			
W	**Recovery run** 45:00 Z1	Water, water + electrolytes, or nothing	At least 0.4 g CHO, 0.1 g PRO per kg body weight	Day 3 of reduced calorie intake Day 3 of 10-day fat-loading period (65 percent of calories from fat) (optional)
T	**Foundation run** 5:00 Z1 35:00 Z2 5:00 Z1	Water, water + electrolytes, or nothing	At least 0.4 g CHO, 0.1 g PRO per kg body weight	Day 4 of reduced calorie intake Day 4 of 10-day fat-loading period (65 percent of calories from fat) (optional)
F	**Tempo run** 5:00 Z1 10:00 Z2 30:00 Z3 10:00 Z2 5:00 Z1	Water, water + electrolytes, or nothing	At least 0.8 g CHO, 0.2 g PRO per kg body weight	Day 5 of reduced calorie intake Day 5 of 10-day fat-loading period (65 percent of calories from fat) (optional)
S	**Recovery run** 45:00 Z1	Water, water + electrolytes, or nothing	At least 0.4 g CHO, 0.1 g PRO per kg body weight	Day 6 of reduced calorie intake Day 6 of 10-day fat-loading period (65 percent of calories from fat) (optional)
S	**Long run with fast finish** 0.5 mile Z1 11.5 miles Z2 1.0 mile Z3	Sports drink or gels + water	At least 0.8 g CHO, 0.2 g PRO per kg body weight	Day 7 of reduced calorie intake Start 7-day caffeine fast (optional) Day 7 of 10-day fat-loading period (65 percent of calories from fat) (optional)

LEVEL 3 / WEEK 20 / TAPER PERIOD				
	WORKOUT	NUTRITION DURING WORKOUT	RECOVERY NUTRITION (WITHIN 45:00 OF COMPLETING WORKOUT)	GENERAL DIET
M	**Recovery run** 45:00 Z1	Water, water + electrolytes, or nothing	At least 0.4 g CHO, 0.1 g PRO per kg body weight	Day 8 of reduced calorie intake Day 8 of 10-day fat-loading period (65 percent of calories from fat) (optional) OR Start 5-day fat-loading period (optional) Day 2 of 7-day caffeine fast (optional)
T	**Speed-play run** 5:00 Z1 10:00 Z2 8 × (0:30 Z4/ 2:30 Z2) 5:00 Z1	Water, water + electrolytes, or nothing	At least 0.4 g CHO, 0.1 g PRO per kg body weight	Day 9 of reduced calorie intake Day 9 of 10-day fat-loading period (65 percent of calories from fat) (optional) OR Day 2 of 5-day fat-loading period (optional) Day 3 of 7-day caffeine fast (optional)
W	**Recovery run** 45:00 Z1	Water, water + electrolytes, or nothing	At least 0.4 g CHO, 0.1 g PRO per kg body weight	Day 10 of reduced calorie intake Day 10 of 10-day fat-loading period (65 percent of calories from fat) (optional) OR Day 3 of 5-day fat-loading period (optional) Day 4 of 7-day caffeine fast (optional)
T	**Fast-finish run** 5:00 Z1 20:00 Z2 10:00 Z3	Water, water + electrolytes, or nothing	At least 0.4 g CHO, 0.1 g PRO per kg body weight	Day 11 of reduced calorie intake Day 1 of 3-day carbo-loading period (70 percent of calories from CHO) OR Day 4 of 5-day fat-loading period (optional) Day 5 of 7-day caffeine fast (optional)

		LEVEL 3 / WEEK 20 / TAPER PERIOD / CONTINUED		
	WORKOUT	NUTRITION DURING WORKOUT	RECOVERY NUTRITION (WITHIN 45:00 OF COMPLETING WORKOUT)	GENERAL DIET
F	**Recovery run** 30:00 Z1	Water, water + electrolytes, or nothing	At least 0.4 g CHO, 0.1 g PRO per kg body weight	Day 12 of reduced calorie intake Day 2 of 3-day carbo-loading period (70 percent of calories from CHO) OR Day 5 of 5-day fat-loading period (optional) Day 6 of 7-day caffeine fast (optional)
S	**Speed-play run** 5:00 Z1 5:00 Z2 4 × (0:30 Z4/ 1:30 Z2) 5:00 Z1	Water, water + electrolytes, or nothing	At least 0.4 g CHO, 0.1 g PRO per kg body weight	Day 3 of 3-day carbo-loading period (70 percent of calories from CHO) OR Day 1 of 1-day carbo-loading period (10 g CHO per kg body weight) (optional) Day 7 of 7-day caffeine fast (optional)
S	**Marathon**	Race nutrition plan	Anything you want!	Prerace nutrition plan

ACKNOWLEDGMENTS

I wish to express my heartfelt thanks to the following men and women who made this book both possible and better than I could have made it alone: Iris Bass, Kevin Beck, Rochelle Cuff, Desiree Davila, Christine Dore, Fred Dufner, Anthony Famiglietti, Nataki Fitzgerald, Sean Fitzgerald, Shalane Flanagan, Mario Fraioli, Gabriel Gastelum, Brett Gotcher, Kara Goucher, Ryan Hall, Kevin Hanover, John Heusner, Libbie Hickman, Asker Jeukendrup, Scott Jurek, Deena Kastor, Meb Keflezighi, Linda Konner, Joe Lemel, Annie Lenth, Irit Levy, David Morken, Kim Mueller, Dave Munger, T.J. Murphy, Tim Noakes, Kate Percy, Robert Portman, Ben Rapoport, Kristian Rauhala, Pete Rea, Dathan Ritzenhein, Stephanie Rothstein, Jonathan Sainsbury, Mark Sands, Renée Sedliar, and Ross Tucker.

APPENDIX: TRAINING AND NUTRITION JOURNAL

Here's an example of a log for your training and nutrition as you prepare for your next marathon or half marathon. Photocopy or scan this to create your own personalized log for as many weeks as you plan on training. (Note that while you will probably find it easiest to keep a running tally of the food types you eat throughout the week, it is only the totals at the end of the week that are important.)

DATE RANGE: _____

TRAINING	
MONDAY	
TUESDAY	
WEDNESDAY	
THURSDAY	
FRIDAY	
SATURDAY	
SUNDAY	
TOTALS:	

DIET	
FOOD TYPE	**NUMBER OF TIMES EATEN**
Vegetables	
Fruits	
Nuts and Seeds	
Fish and Lean Meats	
Whole Grains	
Dairy Products	
Refined Grains	
Fatty Meats	
Sweets	
Fried Foods	

INDEX

ABOUT THE AUTHOR

Matt Fitzgerald is a highly respected endurance sports nutritionist, training expert, and writer. His many previous books include *Racing Weight* and *Performance Nutrition for Runners*. Certified by the International Society of Sports Nutrition, Matt has served as a consultant to several sports nutrition companies. He is also a Training Intelligence Specialist for PEAR Sports. A lifelong runner, Matt lives in Northern California with his wife, Nataki.